Materials Management
Policy and Procedure Manual

Second Edition

Jamie C. Kowalski

The views expressed in this publication are strictly those of the author and do not necessarily represent official positions of Kowalski-Dickow Associates, Inc.

Library of Congress Cataloging-in-Publication Data

Kowalski, Jamie C.
   Materials management policy and procedure manual / Jamie C. Kowalski.
      p.   cm.
   ISBN 0-87125-168-X
   1. Hospitals—Materials management.   I. Catholic Health Association of the
   United States.   II. Title.
   [DNLM: 1. Materials Management, Hospital—handbooks. WX 39 K88m]
RA971.33.K68 1989
362.1'1'0687—dcl9
for Library of Congress   89-929
                                                                       CIP

Catalog no. 142100

copyright ©1990 by Jamie C. Kowalski

Printed in the USA

IM—03/94—0373

DEDICATION

This work is dedicated to my wife, Mary, whose support during the long hours it took to put together this manual cannot be measured and can never be repaid. Also to my sons, Jonathan, Peter, and Charlie, I hope that this country will be able to provide them with high-quality, cost-effective healthcare as a result of hospitals utilizing materials management concepts and some of the ideas presented in this manual.

TABLE OF CONTENTS

EXPANDED TABLE OF CONTENTS

XV.   Patient Transportation 439

XVI.   Waste Handling 453

GLOSSARY

cart lift — an elevator-type mechanism that is used to transport carts only; can be automated (with a device that pulls in and/or pushes out carts), or "manual," for which carts must be loaded and unloaded by personnel.

chargeable supply — any product that is chargeable directly to the patient for whom it is used. Charging mechanism is usually a charge ticket or other similar document.

dispatch — that function within materials management/distribution responsible for responding to requests for supplies and coordinating the delivery of scheduled and nonscheduled supply orders. This function might also be responsible for accepting requests for patient transportation or other types of messenger services.

dumbwaiter — a small version of an elevator-type vertical transportation conveyance mechanism; can be used for small item movement between floors.

economic order quantity (EOQ) — a mathematical formula designed to minimize total costs. It determines the quantity of a given supply that should be ordered each time an order is placed. This formula considers order processing costs, storage costs, inventory carrying costs, total usage, and the unit cost of the product(s).

exchange cart system — supply distribution method that uses a mobile cart as the storage and material-handling module. A predetermined quantity (par level) of a variety of supplies is maintained on carts by materials management personnel. The quantities are determined based on the frequency of restocking and the expected usage during the restocking time interval. At restocking time, the cart maintained in the user department is exchanged with a duplicate (twin) cart that is delivered by materials management. The "used" cart is returned to materials management for counting and restocking. This can be done daily, several times a day, several times a week, or as needed.

full-time equivalent (FTE) — a budget staff position that works and is paid for 2,080 hours per year. Any positions that are budgeted to work less than that number of hours are calculated to be less than 1.0 FTE. For example, someone working 1,040 hours per year is a 0.5 FTE (2,808 - 1,040).

inventory control — the process of accounting for inventory items and dollar value. This includes receipt, issue, credit, physical count verification, adjustments, and so on.

inventory management — a program for optimizing the productivity of inventory as a valuable, current asset. The objective is to provide acceptable levels of service/supply continuity while maintaining low investment levels and carrying costs.

lot number — a reference number that identifies a manufacturing process or sterilizer cycle which products must go through before being ready to use. All products that are processed in a given cycle or sterilizer load are assigned the same lot number. This reference number is useful for product recalls or other types of research and evaluation.

materials management — an integrated group of programs, systems, functions, or departments designed to provide the supplies and other materials used to support patient care and institutional operations in a cost-effective manner. The objective is to provide the right item, to the right place, at the right time, for the lowest total cost.

nonchargeable supply — a supply that is not charged to individual patients. The cost is absorbed by or allocated to operations and included as general "overhead."

nonstock items — items not maintained in the storeroom/warehouse, but used exclusively by and stored in user departments. Sometimes called "specials" or "direct department" supplies, these items are not considered as a part of the official "book"/balance sheet inventory.

par restock system — a supply distribution process that is very similar to the exchange cart system. Predetermined quantities of supplies maintained in user departments are established based on expected usage and the restocking frequency (time interval). Inventory levels in user departments can be maintained on carts, in shelves, and in closets. Counting of levels on hand can be completed by user department personnel or materials management. Frequency can be several times a day, daily, several times a week, or weekly. If a par level of 10 for a given item is established, when the levels are checked and 4 remain, 6 are provided to bring the quantity onhand in the user department "up to par."

pneumatic tube system (PTS) — a small item material-handling conveyance mechanism such as that used in drive-in bank windows. A cylindrical container is loaded with the goods to be transported, placed in the station/system, and transported via air power through tubes throughout the facility. Carriers/containers are usually 4"-6" in diameter and approximately 15"-18" long.

purchasing — the process and function responsible for procuring the right goods in a timely manner for the lowest total cost.

space to demand — a storage system whereby space for supplies in a storeroom or warehouse is allocated based on an expected demand/usage rate for a specified period. For example, a one-week supply would be 10 boxes of a given item. Space in the designated storage area for that item is allocated based on providing up to 10 boxes.

sterile processing — the function responsible for the collection, cleaning, decontamination, assembly, packaging, and final sterilization of reusable products: instruments, utensils, linen, equipment, and so on. This includes chemical disinfection, steam and ethylene oxide (ETO) sterilization, and any other acceptable methods.

stock items — items maintained in the perpetual, official inventory account until they are issued and used by departments. Usually these items are maintained in the storeroom/warehouse.

storeroom/warehouse — the facility and operation in which "stock" (official inventory) items are maintained for issue and use by any department throughout the healthcare facility.

supply distribution system — a predetermined method of managing and delivering supplies from the point of storage to the point of use.

supply processing and distribution (SPD) — that division within materials management that is responsible for the processing, storage, and handling/delivery of reusable and disposable products.

SECTION I

MATERIALS MANAGEMENT ADMINISTRATION
SECTION I

Subject	Effective Date 1-90	Latest Revision & Date
MATERIALS MANAGEMENT MISSION AND SCOPE		

Materials management is responsible for the development, maintenance, and coordination of all supply support systems, 24 hours a day, 365 days a year. Materials management's primary objective is to provide continuous supplies by placing the right item, at the right place, at the right time, for the right price (cost to the healthcare institution).

The quality of the services provided is measured by the degree to which space, personnel, equipment, dollars, and time are used efficiently.

The functions combined under materials management are:

1. Purchasing
2. Inventory control
3. Receiving
4. Storage
5. Dispatch/distribution
6. Print shop
7. Mail service
8. Material processing
9. Linen service
10. Patient transportation

Affected Departments

Reviewed _____

Page 1 of 1

MATERIALS MANAGEMENT
ORGANIZATIONAL CHART

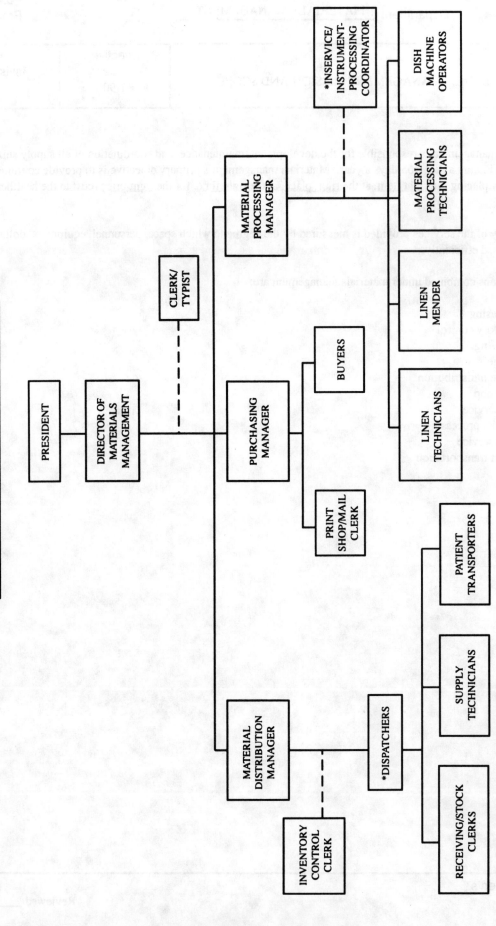

*Functions as the person in charge during manager's absence.

PRESIDENT

DIRECTOR OF MATERIALS MANAGEMENT

CLERK/TYPIST

MATERIAL PROCESSING MANAGER

*INSERVICE/INSTRUMENT-PROCESSING COORDINATOR

DISH MACHINE OPERATORS

MATERIAL PROCESSING TECHNICIANS

LINEN MENDER

LINEN TECHNICIANS

PURCHASING MANAGER

BUYERS

PRINT SHOP/MAIL CLERK

MATERIAL DISTRIBUTION MANAGER

INVENTORY CONTROL CLERK

*DISPATCHERS

PATIENT TRANSPORTERS

SUPPLY TECHNICIANS

RECEIVING/STOCK CLERKS

JOB DESCRIPTION

TITLE: Director of materials management

RESPONSIBLE TO: Senior management

RESPONSIBLE FOR: Developing, implementing. and administering a coordinated supply support system that operates efficiently and meets the needs of the institution's departments. Specifically, this calls for:

Developing policy and procedures in purchasing, inventory control, receiving and storage, distribution, print shop, mail service, material processing, and linen service.

Using personnel, space, equipment, dollars (in purchases and inventory), and time to meet objectives.

Providing administrative support to senior management in the form of reports, budgets, supply utilization analysis, forms management, and capital expenditure management.

Developing department staff through ongoing coaching, inservice education, on-the-job training, and evaluation.

Maintaining good working relationships with all departments by providing service, management assistance, and open communications.

Maintaining adequate operating supply levels in the healthcare facility and coordinating timely supply distribution.

Maintaining a high degree of managerial competence through continuing education or participation in seminars, conventions, and institutes, as well as field trips to other institutions.

EDUCATION: A minimum of a bachelor's degree from an accredited college or university, with emphasis on business administration, economics, or a related field is required. A master's degree is preferred. Experience may be accepted in lieu of a master's degree. Certification in materials management by a professional society is desirable.

EXPERIENCE: Five to seven years' experience in healthcare institution materials management is required. A top-level manager is preferred, but a promotable candidate may be considered.

KNOWLEDGE: Familiarity with and working knowledge of:

• Human relations	• Strategic and operations planning
• Customer service	• Negotiation
• Inventory management	• Procurement
• Manufacturing	• Accounting
• Finance	• Infection control
• Material handling	• Facilities planning
• Industrial/systems engineering	• Marketing
• Computer science	• Transportation

TITLE: Director of materials management (cont.)

ACCOUNTABILITIES:
- Maintain a customer service/satisfaction rating of 88 percent in all functional areas.
- Hold annual budget increases to 85 percent of the rate of inflation.
- Maintain staff productivity at 95 percent of standard.
- Maintain total materials and support labor costs at no more than 17 percent of the facility's total operating budget.
- Identify annual operating cost reductions equal to three times total compensation.
- Maintain inventory accuracy (variance) at 98 percent.

JOB DESCRIPTION

TITLE: Clerk/typist

RESPONSIBLE TO: Director of materials management

RESPONSIBLE FOR: Providing administrative assistance to the director and managers of the materials management staff. Specifically, this calls for:

Acting as a receptionist for visitors and sales representatives; answering and clearing telephone calls; setting up appointments and meetings; maintaining departmental files (personnel, equipment, catalogs, price master); typing for the director and the department (memos, procedures, reports); typing purchase orders and other records; preparing departmental reports using information from the director and managers and other data; assisting in other administrative functions as assigned by the director.

EDUCATION: A high school diploma or the equivalent is required. Some business education is desirable.

EXPERIENCE: Two years' experience in a clerical position is required. Ability to type 80 words per minute is required. Shorthand or dictaphone dictation skills are desirable.

ACCOUNTABILITIES:
- Maintain typing speed at 80 words per minute with an accuracy rate of 97 percent.
- Maintain files current within a one-working-day period.
- Produce departmental reports and correspondence within one working day.

JOB DESCRIPTION

TITLE: Material distribution manager

RESPONSIBLE TO: Director of materials management

RESPONSIBLE FOR: Organizing, operating, and supervising the material distribution area, and all its related functions and systems, in an efficient and effective manner. Specifically, this calls for:

Coordinating central receiving, bulk stores, processed stores, inventory control, dispatch, mail room, archives, and patient transport.

Selecting, developing, supervising, and evaluating department staff; preparing departmental records, reports (financial, personnel); maintaining current written policies and procedures; coordinating with user departments the storage and delivery of supplies and equipment on a scheduled basis; operating an exchange cart system for supplies and linen; operating a Nurserver system on the patient care floors; maintaining accurate records (inventory); working with purchasing to maintain adequate levels of supplies to meet patient care demands; establishing and maintaining quality control standards in the department; assisting in the evaluation of supply/equipment products as needed; controlling patient supply charges and seeing to their proper processing and related functions.

The manager may assist or fill in during the absence of the material processing manager.

Participating in management courses and periodic seminars and institutes will be required.

EDUCATION: A high school diploma or the equivalent and a minimum of two years of college are required. An associate's or bachelor's degree is preferred. Related experience may be accepted in lieu of formal education. Certification in materials management by a professional society is highly desirable.

EXPERIENCE: Four or more years' experience as a supervisor or manager, with progressive responsibility, in a healthcare facility supply area is required. A thorough knowledge of warehousing, inventory control, and modern, healthcare-related material-handling systems is required.

ACCOUNTABILITIES:
- Maintain customer service levels at 90 percent.
- Maintain stock item service levels at 95 percent.
- Maintain productivity levels at 90 percent of standard.
- Maintain error rates at 4 percent of all transactions.

8

JOB DESCRIPTION

TITLE: Inventory control clerk

RESPONSIBLE TO: Material distribution manager

RESPONSIBLE FOR: Maintaining the computer inventory system in a timely and accurate manner. The inventory managed by the system is a very valuable asset. Specifically, this calls for:

Preparing all inventory transactions before submittal to data processing for data entry (master file additions and deletions, daily purchases, receipt and issue transactions, corrections, vendor return credits, returns to stock); batching and line totaling all batches for data entry; logging, filing, and maintaining source documents in an organized fashion; verifying all inventory reports to prove that all information was entered and processed properly; making any corrections to transaction errors after thoroughly researching to find the source of the error; auditing the inventory transactions in purchasing, receiving, or storeroom for accuracy before entry into the system and periodically following processing; taking periodic inventories to prove the accuracy of the system, and preparing corrections and reports for the director of materials management.

Other duties may be assigned by the manager.

EDUCATION: A high school diploma or the equivalent is required. Business education is preferred. Experience may be accepted in lieu of formal training.

EXPERIENCE: One year's experience with an inventory control system is required. Familiarity with and knowledge of medical supplies is highly preferred. Training is provided to orient the experienced person to the institution's specific inventory system.

ACCOUNTABILITIES:
- Maintain records current within four hours of transaction time.
- Maintain accuracy within 98 percent; on-hand count versus file count.
- Produce reports within two working days of request.

JOB DESCRIPTION

TITLE: Dispatcher

RESPONSIBLE TO: Material distribution manager

RESPONSIBLE FOR: Planning, organizing, and controlling material movement throughout the healthcare institution. Specifically, this calls for:

Handling all communications from patient floors and user departments—their supply/equipment requests; scheduling the movement of all exchange carts (supply, linen, food, unit dose); controlling, issuing, and delivering patient care (rental) equipment (including orthopedic, suction machines, etc.); coordinating the use of trash carts and their subsequent allocation/return to assigned areas; setting up emergency surgical case carts; handling emergency, early, or late receivings; controlling patient supply charge tags and equipment charge tickets and coordinating their further processing in the business office and in data processing; maintaining proper inventory records, as required, when filling supply orders; obtaining (STAT) emergency or unusual supplies in coordination with the purchasing department.

Other functions may be assigned by the manager.

The dispatcher also assumes the role of team leader in the absence of the manager.

EDUCATION: A high school diploma or the equivalent is required. Some college is desirable.

EXPERIENCE: Two or more years' experience working with medical supplies and equipment in a healthcare facility is required. This can be in central supply, in an operating room, or on a patient care floor (either in a private or a military institution). Experience with a centralized materials management/exchange cart system is desirable. Ability to comprehend and handle patient charges and inventory documentation is mandatory. Further on-the-job training is provided. Excellent communication skills and ability to establish priorities are required.

ACCOUNTABILITIES:
- Maintain schedule of orders and carts delivered on time.
- Maintain nonscheduled supply order response time of less than 10 minutes.

JOB DESCRIPTION

TITLE: Receiving/stock clerk

RESPONSIBLE TO: Material distribution manager

RESPONSIBLE FOR: Receiving, controlling, storing, and accurately issuing all items stored in inventory (stock). This is generally more than 1,600 different items. Specifically, this calls for:

Receiving, inspecting, verifying, and accepting or rejecting all supplies and equipment delivered to the institution; accurately processing all necessary paperwork/documentation, such as packing slips, bills of lading, receiving reports, control copies, and logs, so that payments can be authorized; preparing all items for return shipment and coordinating this with the user department and with purchasing; accurately preparing and processing all inventory documentation concerned with storage and distribution of supplies, including receipts, receiving reports, stock issue requisitions, return-to-stock credits, returns to vendors, etc.; maintaining neat and accurate files; maintaining a neat, clean work environment and using good storage distribution techniques: proper location, rotation, identification, documentation, and organization; handling and storing sterile supplies to protect the integrity of the sterility; notifying the manager or the purchasing office when supply levels reach reorder points or critically low levels; coordinating the distribution/delivery of supplies (bulk or exchange cart) with the manager, dispatcher, and user department on a scheduled basis; attaching the proper patient charge tag to the respective supplies; inventorying supply exchange; restocking the carts in a neat, orderly fashion; conducting scheduled and random inventories.

Other functions may be assigned by the manager.

EDUCATION: A high school diploma or the equivalent is required.

EXPERIENCE: Previous experience with storage and distribution of supplies is desirable. Knowledge of medical/surgical supplies and equipment will help the clerk be more effective. On-the-job training is provided.

ACCOUNTABILITIES:
- Maintain backlog in receiving of less than one working day.
- Maintain supply issue/delivery schedule; fill and deliver all orders within one working day.
- Maintain record-keeping accuracy at 97 percent.
- Maintain productivity rate at 95 percent of standard.

JOB DESCRIPTION

TITLE: Supply technician

RESPONSIBLE TO: Material distribution manager

RESPONSIBLE FOR: Delivering supplies and equipment to patient care areas efficiently, accurately, and punctually and ultimately returning them for reprocessing or disposal. Specifically, this calls for:

Maintaining adequate supply levels (medical/surgical, pharmacy, linen, etc.) in all patient Nurservers and in other areas (surgery, emergency, pediatrics); coordinating the exchange of all carts (supply, linen, food, unit dose) in the designated areas; handling supplies and equipment to ensure sterility and infection control; controlling the patient care equipment (orthopedic, suction machines, etc.) on the floors assigned—making sure they are available and in working order; coordinating the cleaning of Nurservers and supply utility rooms as scheduled and as needed; controlling patient charges for supplies and equipment issued to patients in the assigned areas; obtaining random (STAT) emergency or unusual supplies with the other materials management personnel; assisting patient care staff with identification of supply needs and available alternatives, when requested.

Other functions may be assigned by the manager.

EDUCATION: A high school diploma or the equivalent is required. Some college is desirable.

EXPERIENCE: Twelve to eighteen months' experience working with patient care supplies and equipment is preferred, either in a central supply, surgery, or patient care area. An ability to communicate well and handle clerical control systems is also required. An understanding of the use/purpose of supplies and equipment is highly desirable. Further on-the-job training is provided. Excellent communication skills are required.

ACCOUNTABILITIES:
• Maintain accuracy at 98 percent of all items prepared.
• Maintain productivity at 95 percent of standard.

JOB DESCRIPTION

TITLE: Purchasing manager

RESPONSIBLE TO: Director of materials management

RESPONSIBLE FOR: Purchasing all supplies, equipment, and services for the healthcare institution. The purchasing manager has the sole authority for committing institutional funds by contract (purchase order). Specifically, this calls for:

Operating, directing, and supervising the purchasing office and its functions; hiring, developing, supervising, and evaluating department personnel; conducting market research, product research, and product evaluation; contacting, negotiating with, and evaluating vendors; negotiating and approving contracts for goods and services; obtaining and reviewing bids from vendors; documenting/authorizing all institutional purchases; maintaining all records pertaining to the purchase of goods and services; verifying and authorizing all invoices for payment; coordinating all product returns; maintaining adequate inventory; preparing departmental reports (financial, personnel, budget, etc.); working with departments to determine needs, establish specifications, review contracts, etc.; attending in-house and outside meetings to keep abreast of product developments, trends, etc., thus maintaining support among the facility's departments and industry peers.

EDUCATION: A bachelor's degree in business administration, economics, or a related field is required. Experience may be accepted in lieu of formal education.

EXPERIENCE: Three to five years in a purchasing department with progressive responsibility is required. Experience with healthcare medical/surgical equipment and supplies is desirable. Excellent communication and negotiation skills are required.

ACCOUNTABILITIES:
- Maintain an average product price index at 95 percent of the medical products price index.
- Maintain fixed price contracts for one year or more on 75 percent of all items purchased.
- Maintain nonstock requisition turnaround time of two working days.
- Maintain group-purchasing use/compliance at 80 percent.

JOB DESCRIPTION

TITLE: Print shop/mail clerk

RESPONSIBLE TO: Purchasing manager

RESPONSIBLE FOR: Handling all in-house printing and copying; maintaining all duplicating/copying equipment; maintaining forms control files; doing some layout/typing. Specifically, this calls for:

Operating copying/duplicating machines, paper cutter, collator, folding machine, mimeograph machine, and small printing press; performing routine maintenance and cleaning of all machines; typing/revising forms as needed/requested; maintaining forms control master file; printing and padding all in-house forms for inventory and single department use; keeping records on machine utilization, maintenance, supply usage, etc.; printing all special requests and publications for use as needed; maintaining adequate supply levels in the print shop; processing all incoming and outgoing mail and distributing when necessary.

Other functions may be assigned by the manager.

EDUCATION: A high school diploma or the equivalent is required.

EXPERIENCE: Good physical condition, clerical aptitude, dependability, cooperation/tact, accuracy, and productivity are required. On-the-job training is provided. Prior experience is not required.

ACCOUNTABILITIES:
- Maintain print requisition turnaround time at three working days.
- Maintain productivity at 95 percent of standard.
- Maintain costs per image produced at the budget/standard rate.

JOB DESCRIPTION

TITLE: Buyer

RESPONSIBLE TO: Purchasing manager

RESPONSIBLE FOR: General processing of purchase orders (both stock and nonstock) for institutional supplies and equipment, as directed by the purchasing manager. Specifically, this calls for:

Communicating by phone with in-house departments and outside vendors; reviewing and updating, as needed, catalogs, price lists, inventory records, files, product/vendor files; clearing vendors for contact/ visits with in-house departments; obtaining prices, quotes, and other product information for user departments; reviewing back-order files and expediting; arranging with other institutions for the lending/borrowing of items, when conditions dictate; coordinating product returns; verifying packing slips against purchase orders for authorization of invoice payment; ordering stock and nonstock supplies; typing purchase orders as necessary, and following up until the item is received, accepted, and paid for; establishing feasible, acceptable delivery dates.

Other functions may be assigned by the purchasing manager.

EDUCATION: An associate's or bachelor's degree in business education is required.

EXPERIENCE: Three years' experience in a purchasing department with progressive responsibility is required. Experience with medical/surgical supplies and equipment is desirable.

ACCOUNTABILITIES:
- Obtain products and services at budgeted prices.
- Maintain competitive opportunities through documented competitive bids on all purchases exceeding $500.
- Maintain group-purchasing contract compliance at 80 percent.

JOB DESCRIPTION

TITLE: Material processing manager

RESPONSIBLE TO: Director of materials management

RESPONSIBLE FOR: Operating, directing, and supervising the material processing area and all its related systems in an efficient, effective manner. Specifically, this calls for:

Coordinating the reprocessing of all supplies and equipment used in the healthcare facility. The processing functions are: decontamination, dishwashing, preparation and packaging, terminal sterilization or sanitization, preparing surgical case cart system and linen packs.

Selecting, developing, supervising, and evaluating department staff; preparing departmental reports and records (financial, budget, personnel, etc.); coordinating with user departments the processing and reassembly of medical supplies, equipment, and instrumentation; maintaining adequate quantities of reprocessed supplies and equipment to meet patient care demands; establishing and maintaining quality control systems as they relate to infection control, sterilizer monitoring, packaging, and processing, etc., in accordance with institutional and departmental policy and regulatory agency requirements; operating all departmental equipment; evaluating products used in production or patient care in the institution; performing other related functions.

The manager may assist or fill in during the absence of the material distribution manager.

Participation in management courses and periodic continuing education programs and seminars is required.

EDUCATION: A bachelor's degree in business or healthcare management is required. Certification as a central supply or operating room technician is required. Related experience may be accepted in lieu of formal education.

EXPERIENCE: Three to five years' experience as a central supply or operating room technician or as a related department manager is required. A thorough knowledge of the following is required: asepsis; surgical techniques, instruments, and equipment; respiratory therapy equipment; and other patient care equipment and supplies and their use. Experience in a centralized processing department and knowledge of related semiautomated systems and equipment are preferred. Medical experience in the military is acceptable.

ACCOUNTABILITIES:
- Maintain an error rate at no more than 2 percent for all items processed and case carts filled.
- Maintain a 0.5 percent positive culture rate on sterilizer cycles.
- Maintain productivity rates at 95 percent of standard.
- Maintain operational costs at budget level.

JOB DESCRIPTION

TITLE: Inservice/instrument-processing coordinator

RESPONSIBLE TO: Material processing manager

RESPONSIBLE FOR: Processing (from decontamination to terminal sterilization) all surgical instruments and returning them to the user department; providing orientation and training to all department personnel through development and implementation of the materials management training program. Specifically, this calls for:

Training instrument-processing technicians in the full scope of their responsibilities; assisting the technicians in processing those instruments; maintaining an adequate level of instruments in circulation and inventorying by control, periodic counts, and reordering (in conjunction with the processing manager and operating room supervisor) when necessary; coordinating the updating of instrument Kardex file, catalog, and reference manuals; maintaining an adequate supply of surgical implants and other specialty supplies and equipment; maintaining accurate records; coordinating programs for further staff development with the surgery inservice instructor, processing manager, and operating room supervisor.

Other duties may be assigned by the manager.

The inservice coordinator also assumes the role of team leader in the absence of the manager.

EDUCATION: An associate's degree is required. Continuing education as a licensed practical nurse or certification as an operating room or central supply technician also is required. A bachelor's degree is desirable.

EXPERIENCE: Three to five years' experience with progressive responsibility in surgery or in a centralized processing department handling surgical instruments is required. Prior instructing experience is desirable. Attendance at management/supervisory development programs will be required for anyone lacking experience as a supervisor.

ACCOUNTABILITIES:
* Maintain departmental productivity and quality standards.
* Maintain a 100 percent success rate for all staff who complete the departmental processing technician training course.
* Maintain at least 25 percent of the staff at a certified technician level.

JOB DESCRIPTION

TITLE: Linen technician

RESPONSIBLE TO: Material processing manager

RESPONSIBLE FOR: Receiving, storing, and distributing clean, processed linen in-house and returning soiled linen to the commercial laundry for reprocessing. Specifically, this calls for:

Setting up packs of linen for the operating room, the emergency room, and the rest of the institution; coordinating, weighing, and recording the weight of all clean linen the facility receives from the commercial laundry; completing necessary paperwork for proper documentation of clean linen processed/received; weighing and packaging of soiled linen before shipment to aid infection control in the facility; setting up all linen exchange or replenishment carts as needed or scheduled; coordinating delivery of the carts with the dispatcher; assisting with calls for emergency or extra linen.

Other functions may be assigned by the manager.

EDUCATION: A high school diploma or the equivalent is preferred. Ability to read and write legibly and understand written and verbal communication is required. Ability to process the necessary paperwork is required.

EXPERIENCE: On-the-job training is provided. No prior experience is necessary.

ACCOUNTABILITIES:
- Deliver all orders on schedule.
- Fill all orders accurately.
- Maintain quality levels by keeping properly prepared packs and clean, lint-free linen at 95 percent.
- Maintain productivity levels at 95 percent of standard.

JOB DESCRIPTION

TITLE: Linen mender

RESPONSIBLE TO: Material processing manager

RESPONSIBLE FOR: Preparing and repairing reprocessable linen items used in the institution. Specifically, this calls for:

Assisting linen pack room personnel when time is available; repairing bed linen, patient gowns, scrub clothing, wrappers, and other linen items used in the institution; making up new covers, wrappers, and other items as requested/directed by the manager; maintaining identifiable emblems (institutional identification) on all new and existing linen; preparing and maintaining adequate cleaning/repair records as required by the department or the manager.

Other functions may be assigned by the manager.

EDUCATION: A high school diploma or the equivalent is preferred. Ability to read and write legibly and understand written and verbal instructions is required.

EXPERIENCE: Experience in operating a sewing machine, surger, heat-seal patcher, and other sewing equipment is required. On-the-job training is provided.

ACCOUNTABILITIES:
- Maintain backlog at no more than three working days.
- Complete special-request orders within five working days.

JOB DESCRIPTION

TITLE: Material processing technician

RESPONSIBLE TO: Material processing manager

RESPONSIBLE FOR: Identifying, disassembling, decontaminating, inspecting, assembling, and processing all reusable supplies and patient care equipment used in the institution. Specifically, this calls for:

Receiving, identifying, and decontaminating more than 500 types of surgical instruments, respiratory therapy equipment, patient care and orthopedic equipment, carts, and other miscellaneous supplies and utensils; inspecting, assembling, wrapping, terminal (steam or ETO gas) sterilizing, storing, and redistributing to user departments; operating all departmental equipment used in the processing system—sonic cleaner, washer/sterilizer, dishwasher, ETO gas sterilizer and aerator, high-vacuum steam sterilizer, impulse heat sealer, cart washer; handling and storage of sterile supplies to ensure the integrity of the sterility and maintain sterile shelf life; setting up and distributing scheduled and emergency surgical case carts; maintaining adequate and accurate sterilizer records that monitor the equipment's operation and effectiveness; maintaining an adequate level of working supplies by notifying the manager or ordering them from the storeroom in the manager's absence (in emergencies); maintaining a neat, clean, safe work environment.

Other functions may be assigned by the manager.

EDUCATION: A high school diploma or the equivalent is required. Successful completion of a program for operating room or central supply technicians is required.

EXPERIENCE: On-the-job training is provided. Prior experience is not required but is preferred.

ACCOUNTABILITIES:
- Maintain productivity at 90 percent of standard.
- Maintain accuracy of instruments and equipment processed at 98 percent (error-free).
- Maintain accuracy of cart picking at 98 percent.
- Maintain negative rate for biological culture results at 99.75 percent.

JOB DESCRIPTION

TITLE: Dish machine operator

RESPONSIBLE TO: Material processing manager

RESPONSIBLE FOR: Operating the dishwashing machine and cleaning and sanitizing all dishware and food utensils. Specifically, this calls for:

Setting up, operating, taking down, and cleaning the dishwashing machine; maintaining the machine; contacting the manager for assistance from maintenance or the manufacturer's service representative in the event of major malfunctions; cleaning walls, floors, and machines daily; transporting utensils to the kitchen after cleaning; hand-washing carts as necessary; assisting in other areas of decontamination as assigned by the manager or when free time is available.

EDUCATION: High school graduation is not required. This position requires the ability to read and write and to understand written and verbal instructions. Ability to communicate verbally is required. Students are acceptable.

EXPERIENCE: No previous experience is required. On-the-job training is provided.

ACCOUNTABILITIES:
- Maintain productivity rate at 95 percent of standard.
- Maintain reject rate at less than 7 percent.

JOB DESCRIPTION

TITLE: Patient transporter

RESPONSIBLE TO: Material distribution manager

RESPONSIBLE FOR: Safe and efficient transport and escort of patients throughout the institution. Specifically, this calls for:

Working with the dispatcher to maintain schedules and establish priorities; establishing rapport with patients and making them feel welcome, secure, and cared for; helping patients into wheelchairs and stretchers; handling patient care equipment and maintaining records of departmental volume and individual transactions.

EDUCATION: High school graduation or equivalent is required. Ability to communicate verbally and maintain records is required. Ability to complete an in-house training program that includes hygiene, first aid, body mechanics, equipment handling, and asepsis is required.

EXPERIENCE: No previous experience is required. This is an entry level position that requires completion of a hospital training program.

ACCOUNTABILITIES:
- Maintain a response rate for patient transport requests at less than 8 minutes.
- Maintain a productivity rate of 75 percent of standard.
- Maintain an incident-free transaction record for six consecutive months, with no more than one incident in a calendar year.
- Maintain accurately timely records of departmental activity.

Subject	Effective Date 1-90	Latest Revision & Date
DRESS CODE		

Materials management personnel are required to adhere to institutional and departmental dress code policy. A positive, professional image should be promoted.

Materials management personnel must always be in uniform while on duty. Failure to comply may result in the employee's being sent home (on his or her time) to change into proper attire.

Uniforms for all processing personnel (processing, decontamination, dishwashing, laundry, linen pack room) consist of complete scrub attire (dresses, or shirts and pants) plus caps to cover the hair. Personnel in decontamination must also wear gloves while working (as should dishwashing personnel). Proper rubber- or crepe-soled shoes should be worn. All processing personnel must wear shoe covers while on duty or a pair of shoes that are worn only on the job. Platform, other high-heeled, or open-toed shoes are not allowed. Scrub clothing is provided by, and laundered by, the institution.

When leaving the work area, decontamination and dishwashing personnel must change into clean scrub clothing and put on lab coats (buttoned up the front).

Other processing personnel will wear buttoned-up lab coats over their scrub attire whenever leaving the work area. They are required to change clothing only at the end of the work day.

Visitors are required to wear scrub clothing or a surgical gown and proper shoe covers and cap when entering the work area. There are no exceptions. The required clothing is discarded in the nearest hamper when the visitor leaves that work area.

Uniforms for distribution personnel (dispatchers, stock clerks, receiving clerks, control clerks, supply technicians) consist of a blue smock jacket worn with white or blue slacks or skirt. No denim jeans are allowed. The smock may be worn with or without a shirt, blouse, or sweater underneath. The smock, which should be laundered regularly by the employee, is purchased by the employee.

Uniform-type shoes are not required, but high-heeled, platform, or open-toed shoes are not allowed. Shoes should have a rubber or crepe sole to provide traction and support on waxed surfaces.

Purchasing and office personnel must follow the institution's dress code.

Name tags must be worn whenever the employee is on duty.

Affected Departments

Reviewed _____

Page 1 of 1

Subject	Effective Date	Latest Revision & Date
DEPARTMENT SECURITY	1-90	

Materials management is staffed 24 hours a day, 7 days a week.

Materials management areas are off-limits to everyone but materials management personnel, except in the case of official business. Requests to enter the department are made through the dispatch office.

Visitors are not allowed to go through the department without an escort from the materials management staff or a security guard.

The following doors are kept locked at or during the times listed:

1. Double doors to dispatch: locked at all times
2. Dispatch restroom door: locked at all times
3. Double doors to decontamination area: locked from 5P.M. to 6A.M.
4. Door to decontamination locker room entrance: locked from 11P.M. to 6A.M.
5. Door inside decontamination area: slide bolt locked from 7P.M. to 11P.M.
6. Door to dishwashing from kitchen: slide bolt locked from 7P.M. to 7A.M. (or when dishwashing crew leaves for the evening)
7. Double doors to bulk stores: locked from 5P.M. to 6A.M.
8. Single door to receiving/stores (near scale): locked from 5P.M. to 6A.M.
9. Linen pack room door: locked at all times
10. Door to compactor: locked at all times
11. Receiving doors: locked at all times
12. Mail/hold room door: locked from 4P.M. to 7A.M.
13. Flammable storage door: locked at all times
14. Pressurized gas storage door: locked at all times
15. Internal door to print shop: locked from 5P.M. to 7A.M. (and whenever the print shop is not staffed)
16. External door to print shop: locked from 5P.M. to 7A.M.
17. Purchasing office doors: locked from 5P.M. to 7A.M.
18. Equipment storage doors: locked at all times
19. Pharmacy doors: locked at all times

The dispatch office and security guards must make sure that the above schedule is followed.

The dispatch office is responsible for the keys to the following areas:

1. Area master for materials management
2. Equipment stores
3. Mail room
4. Cart lifts
5. Mechanical equipment room (second floor)
6. Flammable stores

Affected Departments

Reviewed _____

Subject	Effective Date	Latest Revision & Date
DEPARTMENT SECURITY (cont.)	1-90	

Keys are located in the dispatch office on the key ring. Anyone requesting to use the keys must sign them <u>out</u> in the key log (notebook), kept in the dispatch office, and sign them in again on return.

Keys may be given only to members of materials management or administration. Other personnel will be escorted through the area by a dispatcher or security guard.

The dispatch area should be staffed <u>at all times</u>. If the area must be left vacant, the doors will be locked and the keys taken by the dispatcher. (This includes the entire key ring. Keys should <u>never</u> be removed from the ring.)

Personnel seeking access to materials management during the dispatcher's infrequent absences may page the dispatcher or the security guard and wait for his or her return.

Any unusual occurrences should be noted in the communication book and reported to the security guard. An incident report will be made out by the distribution manager the next working day.

Affected Departments

Reviewed _____

Subject	Effective Date 1-90	Latest Revision & Date
DEPARTMENT SAFETY/INCIDENT REPORTS		

Both employer and employees are responsible for maintaining a clean, neat, and safe institutional environment so that patients, visitors, and employees are not subjected to environmental safety hazards.

When employees become aware of an unsafe condition (wet spill on the floor, improperly placed objects—ladders, hoses, stacked boxes, etc.), they should report it to their immediate supervisor for correction. In the meantime, employees should do what they can either to correct the situation or to stand by so that other persons, unaware of the condition, are not endangered or injured.

If an injury occurs, no matter how insignificant it may seem, the incident should be reported to a manager immediately. This is to protect the employee and the institution legally and physically.

The manager should direct the injured employee to the employee health nurse or the emergency department for examination by a physician. The manager should also obtain and complete an incident report and submit it to the director with a complete account of the incident and any consequences (lost time, corrective measures taken, etc.). The director will investigate and take appropriate steps to eliminate the condition or factor that led to the incident.

Affected Departments

Reviewed _____

Subject	Effective Date	Latest Revision & Date
STAFF SCHEDULING	1-90	

Materials management is open 24 hours a day, 7 days a week. Schedules for materials management will be posted on the bulletin board at the beginning of the last week of each month. Unless there are holidays, vacations, or leaves of absence (LOA), the schedules will be the same each month.

Requests for changes, off days, holidays, etc., must be submitted to the appropriate supervisor, in writing, before the schedule is posted. Emergencies or exceptions will be handled individually. Only a manager may approve any changes, switching, etc.

Several shifts/schedules are assigned to meet departmental demands. These will be explained by the work area's manager.

Affected Departments

Reviewed _____

TIME SCHEDULE

EMPLOYEE'S NAME

POSITION

DEPARTMENT

DEPARTMENT (COST CENTER) NUMBER

REQUEST FOR VACATION/HOLIDAY/APPROVED ABSENCE

DATE _____

EMPLOYEE NAME _____ DEPARTMENT _____

REQUEST FOR ☐ VACATION ☐ HOLIDAY ☐ SPECIAL DAY(S) OFF

VACATION

TOTAL VACATION DAYS DUE _____ ☐ VERIFIED ☐ ADJUSTED _____

TOTAL VACATION DAYS REQUESTED _____

DATE(S) REQUESTED (1st Choice) FROM _____ TO _____

(2nd Choice) FROM _____ TO _____

(3rd Choice) FROM _____ TO _____

(4th Choice) FROM _____ TO _____

HOLIDAY

☐ SPRING HOLIDAY/DATE REQUESTED _____

☐ BIRTHDAY HOLIDAY/DATE REQUESTED _____

☐ OTHER _____ DATE REQUESTED _____
(EXPLAIN)

NON-PAID DAY(S) OFF

TOTAL DAY(S) REQUESTED _____

DATE(S) REQUESTED _____

REASON _____

_____

_____
(EMPLOYEE SIGNATURE)

☐ APPROVED   ☐ APPROVED
☐ NOT APPROVED   ☐ NOT APPROVED

_____   _____   _____   _____
(SUPERVISOR)   (DATE)   (DEPARTMENT HEAD)   (DATE)

Subject	Effective Date 1-90	Latest Revision & Date
PERSONAL VISITORS AND TOURS		

The materials management department and its work areas are restricted to materials management staff only.

Employees from other departments are allowed only for official business.

Personal visitors are not allowed in the department without prior approval of the director.

Employees may meet visitors in the cafeteria or the snack bar (during proper visitor hours) when on a scheduled, approved break.

Personal visitors include employees who are off duty or on vacation days. They are not to linger in the department or work areas to visit with those employees on duty.

All tour requests must be approved in advance by the director and community relations department.

Affected Departments

Reviewed _____

Subject	Effective Date	Latest Revision & Date
EMERGENCIES	1-90	

EXTERNAL DISASTER PLAN

On the announcement of "First Floor Alert," the following procedure will be initiated:

1. The director will report to the control center (nursing service office) to obtain information regarding the number of persons involved, the nature of the disaster, what types of injuries, and what supplies will be needed.

   a. If the director is not on duty, the designated person in charge will report to the control center (the distribution manager, then the processing manager, then the purchasing manager).

   b. If the alert is called on an evening, night, or weekend, the director will be notified at home by the materials management person in charge. (If the director is unavailable, notify the manager on call.)

   c. The materials management person in charge will then begin implementing the alert plan for the materials management department.

2. All materials management employees will return to the department for assignments.

   a. If the alert occurs on an evening, night, or weekend, extra staff will be called in by the appropriate manager with the employees who live closest to the hospital being called in first.

   (1) The purchasing manager will report to obtain any emergency supplies from outside sources.

   (2) The processing manager and a minimum of three technicians will make up linen carts and set up and process instrument sets and equipment.

   (3) The distribution manager and a minimum of three dispatchers or technicians will make up supply carts and transport them to the emergency or operating rooms.

3. Off-duty personnel arriving through the employee entrance should be prepared to present their identification cards to the appropriate authorities. No one must be admitted to the building without this identification.

Affected Departments

Reviewed _____

Subject	Effective Date 1-90	Latest Revision & Date
EMERGENCIES (cont.)		

EXTERNAL DISASTER PLAN (cont.)

4. Specific materials management assignments are:

   a. Dispatchers and stock clerks will immediately restock the emergency room backup supply carts completely and send them to the first-floor clean hold room. The linen cart should also be sent.

   b. Processing technicians will set up the emergency room linen cart for dispatching to the first floor. They will stand by for instructions on any other items to be processed.

   c. The supply technician assigned to the first floor that day will report to the clean hold room and transport the carts sent from dispatch to the corridor between the emergency room and cardiac diagnostics. That supply technician will remain in the emergency room to observe supply needs and obtain them from dispatch as necessary. All supplies are sent on carts by the cart lift (or staff elevator if the lift is not working). All other supply technicians will remain in their assigned areas (patient care floors) and resume routine assignments.

   d. The purchasing staff will stand by to obtain emergency supplies.

   e. All other materials management employees will continue with the usual routine unless instructed otherwise by the director or manager in charge. Telephones should be used only for emergency purposes during the alert.

5. All employees will remain on duty until dismissed by the director or manager in charge.

Affected Departments

Reviewed _____

Subject EMERGENCIES (cont.)	Effective Date 1-90	Latest Revision & Date

CODE BLUE

Materials management employees should be aware of a "code blue" being announced over the public address system. A code blue is called when a patient becomes critically ill (having a cardiac or respiratory arrest).

Supply technicians assigned to the area in which the code occurs should report to the code area in case they are needed to obtain emergency supplies or equipment. They should remember not to get in the way of the lifesaving code team.

Other materials management personnel should not attempt to go near the code area unless requested by a nursing supervisor or a materials management manager.

The dispatchers should remain by the telephone, avoid making any outgoing calls, keep the lines clear, and respond quickly to any requests from the code area.

Affected Departments

Reviewed _____

Subject	Effective Date 1-90	Latest Revision & Date
CARE OF PATIENT IN ISOLATION		

OBTAINING SUPPLIES AND NOTIFICATION OF ISOLATION

1. The nurse will request a specific isolation cart setup (according to the type of isolation) from the administrative communications clerk (ACC).

   The clerk will contact the supply technician, if working, or the dispatcher in materials management. If the ACC is not on duty, the nurse will call the dispatcher directly.

2. The dispatcher will call the ACC and advise that the cart is coming. On night shifts, the dispatcher will notify the nurse in charge.

3. The supply technician on the floor will deliver the cart to the alcove of the patient's room and notify the nurse that the cart has arrived. On evening and night shifts, personnel will be instructed to pick up the isolation cart from the clean hold room.

4. When the supplies come to the floor, the ACC stamps the patient's name on the charge tag that comes with the supplies. This charge tag is returned to materials management.

5. The supply technician will restock the cart every 24 hours. Some additional supplies will be on the cart in the clean hold room. If there are none there, the ACC should contact the supply technician or the dispatcher.

   Additional supplies or increases also can be noted on the control/anticipation sheet for the next day. These must be noted by noon for a 3:30P.M. delivery.

Affected Departments

Reviewed _____

Subject	Effective Date	Latest Revision & Date
CARE OF PATIENT IN ISOLATION (cont.)	1-90	

CARE OF ITEMS IN THE ROOM WHEN ISOLATION IS DISCONTINUED OR WHEN ITEMS ARE REMOVED FROM THE ROOM

Steps	Key Points
1. Discard all paper articles.	Wear protective garb; gloves, mask, etc.
2. Use plastic bags to return supplies to materials management. Bags are available in two sizes, with the word "contaminated" on the outside. They are in the isolation cart.	All articles in the isolation cart, outside the patient's room, are considered clean and may be sent back to materials management for a refund.
3. Separate articles according to the method of sterilization, as follows:	
a. <u>Steam sterilizer</u> Metal dressing trays, instruments, metal basins, bedpans, and any other metal or glass objects go in one bag.	Empty ash trays and wipe clean. Bag plastic glasses loosely and send to materials management to be decontaminated before returning them to the kitchen.
b. <u>Gas sterilizer</u> Sphygmomanometer and stethoscope must be bagged separately. <u>All</u> plastic items may be bagged together.	

Affected Departments

Reviewed _____

Subject		Effective Date 1-90	Latest Revision & Date
CARE OF PATIENT IN ISOLATION (cont.)			

PROCEDURE FOR REMOVING ITEMS FROM ROOM

1. One person stands outside the patient's door with bags marked "contaminated."

A large cuff is made on the bag to protect the hands of the bag handler while articles are being placed in it.

2. Articles are placed in the bags as directed, and the bags are secured with a twist tie.

Bags are closed at the top to prevent exposure to the contaminated portion.

3. Wastebaskets are left in the room to be cleaned and returned to materials management by the housekeeping unit aides.

4. Nondisposable dressing trays are dismantled and bagged as necessary, then placed in the soiled portion of the Nurserver. Soiled instruments should be rinsed before bagging.

Any articles not taken into the patient's room may be returned to materials management with a note indicating that they were not in the contaminated room.

5. All items such as K-pads, weights, portable IV standards, cradles, and machines must be wiped off with disinfectant before being returned to materials management.

6. A clean cloth towel or sheet is placed on a surface in the room to provide a clean space for wiped items.

7. Basin and disinfectant are obtained from the janitor's soiled hold room.

8. Mobile equipment is placed near the door of the room, with paper toweling under each wheel. Wheels are cleaned with disinfectant before the equipment is removed. Items are covered with a large plastic bag labeled "contaminated" or with a sheet labeled "isolation."

9. All large items are taken to the soiled hold room to be returned to materials management by the supply technician. Small items are placed in the soiled portion of the Nurserver.

10. If the patient is discharged, bedpans, emesis basins, wash basins, and urinals must be rinsed free of protein material with diverter valve in bathroom and bagged by the housekeeper. (If the patient remains in the hospital, nursing handles the utensils.)

11. Any unused materials on isolation carts are returned to materials management. The ACC will inform housekeeping that the patient is leaving.

Affected Departments

Reviewed _____

Subject	Effective Date	Latest Revision & Date
QUALITY ASSURANCE AUDIT	1-90	

The quality assurance audit for materials management was developed from departmental objectives. Materials management is responsible for the timely and proper purchase, storage, processing, distribution, and control of all institutional supplies and equipment.

Once this objective was defined, the criteria (Sections I through VII) that should be met by materials management were established. These criteria will indicate how well departmental objectives are being met. In Section VIII, the judgment of the departments being serviced is used as an additional measure of quality.

This survey is conducted and reviewed quarterly by the director. The "yes" answers in the index indicate adherence. The "yes" and "no" answers are tabulated. The percentage of "yes" answers is calculated and the results are graphed so that quality adherence trends can be noted easily.

The results are discussed with the department managers and staff. Then any necessary corrective action is taken. The surveys are maintained in a file for review and follow-up.

Affected Departments

Reviewed _____

Subject	Effective Date 1-90	Latest Revision & Date
QUALITY ASSURANCE AUDIT (cont.)		

I. <u>PURCHASING</u>   <u>YES</u>   <u>NO</u>

   A. Is the purchasing office controlling purchase orders?   _____   _____

   B. Are requisitions processed within two days of receipt or
      the need identified?   _____   _____

   C. Have at least three (3) <u>competitive bids</u> been obtained
      for any orders of $500 or more?   _____   _____

   D. Are there any incomplete or back-ordered purchase orders
      over three (3) months old?   _____   _____

   E. Do purchasing practices take advantage of economical-order
      and price-break quantities?   _____   _____

   F. Are purchase orders consolidated so that line items per purchase
      order exceed back orders?   _____   _____

   G. Are any other departments ordering from vendors?   _____   _____

   H. Is the product evaluation committee meeting objectives?   _____   _____

II. <u>INVENTORY CONTROL</u>

   A. Are stock-outs less than 6 percent?   _____   _____

   B. Are <u>inventory</u> levels as low as possible, short of jeopardizing
      continuity of supplies?   _____   _____

   C. Has the number of line items in inventory increased?   _____   _____

   D. Has the value of the inventory increased?   _____   _____

   E. Is the inventory accurate with 5 percent (on the shelf vs. records)?   _____   _____

   F. Have all inventory documents been processed each day?   _____   _____

   G. Have errors been corrected and reprocessed before the close
      of the period?   _____   _____

   H. Do errors exceed 5 percent of total transactions?   _____   _____

   I. Is annual inventory turnover at least 15 times per year?   _____   _____

Affected Departments

Reviewed _____

Subject	Effective Date 1-90	Latest Revision & Date
QUALITY ASSURANCE AUDIT (cont.)		

III. <u>CHARGES</u>   <u>YES</u>   <u>NO</u>

    A. Have all patient charge tags been processed on time?   _____ _____

    B. Have lost charges been investigated and documented?   _____ _____

    C. Is the total value of the lost charges for the month less than 5 percent
       of total revenue?   _____ _____

    D. Are supply charges based on current costs?   _____ _____

    E. Are total charges lost less than 5 percent of total volume?   _____ _____

    F. Do charge credits exceed 2 percent of total volume?   _____ _____

    G. Have all rental equipment charges been processed at the
       end of the month closing?   _____ _____

IV. <u>PROCESSING</u>

    A. Decontamination

       1. Is the work area clean?   _____ _____

       2. Is processing equipment operating properly?   _____ _____

       3. Are soiled items being handled properly?   _____ _____

       4. Are employees properly attired (scrub clothes, masks,
          caps, gloves)?   _____ _____

       5. Are all items processed before the end of the work day?   _____ _____

    B. Dishwashing

       1. Is work area clean?   _____ _____

       2. Are dishes clean after processing?   _____ _____

       3. Are all microbiology culture results acceptable?   _____ _____

       4. Is equipment working properly?   _____ _____

Affected Departments

Reviewed _____

Subject	Effective Date 1-90	Latest Revision & Date
QUALITY ASSURANCE AUDIT (cont.)		

IV. PROCESSING (cont.)   YES   NO

    C. Preparation/packaging and sterilization

        1. Is work area clean?   _____   _____

        2. Are employees properly attired?   _____   _____

        3. Is the environment acceptable (humidity 40-60 percent,
            temperature 65-80°F)?   _____   _____

        4. Are items being wrapped properly?   _____   _____

        5. Are instrument trays set up properly? (Select one at random and
            check for: proper instruments, proper sequence/setup, instruments
            clean and working, proper handling.)   _____   _____

        6. Is the error rate less than 2 percent?   _____   _____

        7. Do items processed have expiration and sterilization dates?   _____   _____

        8. Are sterilizer monitor record cards up-to-date and accurate? _____   _____

        9. Are microbiology culture results negative?   _____   _____

      10. Is all ETO gas sterilizing centralized with proper exhaust and
           monitoring facilities?   _____   _____

    D. Case carts

        1. Are sterile stores shelves labeled, stocked, and rotated?   _____   _____

        2. Are items within expiration date?   _____   _____

        3. Are case carts filled properly? (Inspect two at random.)   _____   _____

        4. Are all carts prepared for 8P.M. delivery?   _____   _____

        5. Is the emergency cart filled and available?   _____   _____

        6. Are case cart requisitions properly filed?   _____   _____

        7. Is the error rate less than 2 percent?   _____   _____

Affected Departments

Reviewed _____

Subject	Effective Date 1-90	Latest Revision & Date
QUALITY ASSURANCE AUDIT (cont.)		

	YES	NO
V. RECEIVING, STORAGE, AND DISTRIBUTION		
A. Are all items reccived, inspected, and processed on the same day?	_____	_____
B. Are supplies stored in the proper location?	_____	_____
C. Do all stock items have date received and stock number visibly located on them?	_____	_____
D. Are oldest items in position to be used first?	_____	_____
E. Is storeroom neat and clean?	_____	_____
F. Are exchange carts properly organized?	_____	_____
G. Do carts have the proper items and quantities on them?	_____	_____
H. Are carts ready to be delivered at the designated time?	_____	_____
I. Are Nurservers properly stocked? (Select one from each floor at random.)	_____	_____
J. Do errors exceed 5 percent of transactions?	_____	_____
K. Have random calls increased during the month? (Check dispatch log.)	_____	_____
VI. LINEN		
A. Is linen inventory/supply adequate to supply all user departments?	_____	_____
B. Is clean linen received from the commercial laundry clean, pressed, and folded properly?	_____	_____
C. Are linen records up-to-date and accurate (soiled linen sent out, clean linen received, linen sent to departments)?	_____	_____
D. Are microbiology culture records from an independent laboratory available, and have negative results been obtained?	_____	_____
E. Are linen carts clean and working properly?	_____	_____
F. Are cart covers being used in transport and storage?	_____	_____
G. Does linen used/processed exceed 12 pounds (clean) per patient per day?	_____	_____

Affected Departments

Reviewed _____

Subject	Effective Date 1-90	Latest Revision & Date
QUALITY ASSURANCE AUDIT (cont.)		

VII. <u>PRINTING</u>   <u>YES</u>   <u>NO</u>

    A. Have all special orders been filled within the designated time?   _____   _____

    B. Is all equipment working properly?   _____   _____

    C. Are records/files current, with samples of all in-house forms available? _____   _____

    D. Are all forms printed in-house, if possible?   _____   _____

    E. Are log sheets or meters being properly used to show departmental use?   _____   _____

VIII. <u>MISCELLANEOUS</u>

    A. Are written policies and procedures current and available for use in
       materials management and user departments?   _____   _____

    B. Are department schedules posted?   _____   _____

    C. Are communications posted?   _____   _____

    D. Is department physically clean?   _____   _____

    E. Is departmental traffic/security being controlled and monitored?   _____   _____

    F. Are employees properly attired?   _____   _____

    G. Have all employees participated in the orientation/training program?   _____   _____

    H. Are user departments satisfied with response and service?   _____   _____

    I. Is department operating within its budget?   _____   _____

Affected Departments

Reviewed _____

Subject	Effective Date 1-90	Latest Revision & Date
DEPARTMENTAL COMMUNICATIONS		

Daily changes, notices, and important information are noted in the communication book. This spiral notebook is filled out each day by the manager, or person in charge, to inform all staff members about what is going on.

Messages in the communication book should be clear and concise. The person writing the note should sign his or her name after it.

Staff members should read the book each day when they arrive at work.

Calls from staff members calling in sick will be noted in the communication book.

The large bulletin board at the entrance to the department serves as the main communications vehicle for staff members.

All official notices, memos, minutes of meetings, procedures, policies, etc., will be posted on the board for 10 days. Notices will be removed and filed after each employee has initialed the memo to designate that he or she read it.

Personnel should consult the bulletin board daily for important information concerning institutional or departmental changes, activities, etc. Those desiring to place something on the bulletin board should obtain the director's approval.

Written communications, both interdepartmental and intradepartmental, must be approved by the director.

Monthly departmental meetings must be attended by all department personnel. Minutes will be posted on the bulletin board for the specified time.

Affected Departments

Reviewed _____

Subject	Effective Date 1-90	Latest Revision & Date
BUDGETS		

The materials management department, and the entire healthcare institution, must work within an established annual budget.

Budgets, developed according to the institution's service-level needs, are submitted for administrative approval. Once approval is obtained, the budget guidelines are adhered to. Evaluation of management's performance takes budget performance fully into account. All variances must be fully justified and approved.

All expenses (labor, supplies, equipment, repairs, etc.) are budgeted for and are charged to specific budget accounts.

Budget (cost center) accounts
651 Purchasing
652 Material processing
653 Material distribution
654 Linen service
655 Print shop
656 Mail room

Expense account numbers
26 Salaries and wages
37 Office supplies
38 Copy machine expense
39 Postage
41 Institutes, workshops, seminars, and travel
42 Membership dues and subscriptions
53 Linen, bedding, surgical draperies
54 Oxygen and other gases
55 Drugs
56 Intravenous solutions and supplies—stock
57 Intravenous solutions and supplies—nonstock
58 Dressings—stock
59 Dressings—nonstock
60 Instruments
61 Sutures—stock
62 Sutures—nonstock
63 Gloves—stock
64 Gloves—nonstock
65 Specimen containers
66 Needles and syringes—stock
67 Needles and syringes—nonstock
68 Tubing—stock
69 Tubing—nonstock
70 Leasing and rental expense
80 Repairs and maintenance—general
90 Miscellaneous supplies and expenses

Affected Departments

Reviewed _____

Subject	Effective Date	Latest Revision & Date
DEPARTMENTAL PURCHASES	1-90	

All items used by the department must be charged to a budget account.

The department requires supplies to operate on a daily basis. To obtain these supplies:

1. Ask the supervisor to prepare or approve a stock requisition for the item(s) required if it is in inventory. Forward the requisition to the stock clerks for filling and delivery. Acknowledge receipt of the good(s).

2. If the item is to be purchased directly from an outside vendor, the manager should submit a requisition to the director. If approved, the requisition is forwarded to purchasing. On receiving the item(s), receiving will present it (them) to the manager for verification and disposition.

Affected Departments

Reviewed _____

Subject	Effective Date 1-90	Latest Revision & Date
COST CONTAINMENT		

All materials management personnel are responsible for helping the department operate within budget. This can be done by following all procedures that relate to labor or supply use, as required.

In addition, suggestions for achieving cost savings in the department and the institution are encouraged. Suggestions should be detailed and signed so that credit can be given for good ideas. A response will be made to all suggestions, whether implemented or not.

If the employee requests, a manager will assist with the preparation of a formal, written cost-containment suggestion.

Affected Departments

Reviewed _____

Subject		Effective Date	Latest Revision & Date
INSERVICE EDUCATION/ORIENTATION		1-90	

New employees in materials management will receive a formal orientation:

1. To the institution by the personnel department; one half day

2. To their department by their manager; one day

3. To their job by their manager and their "buddy." They will work along with an experienced staff member (buddy) for up to two weeks.

In addition, materials management provides for and requires completion of a one-week training course. The course includes lectures, demonstrations, audiovisuals, and some on-the-job applications. Participants in the course are given written tests to measure their progress and the effectiveness of the program and the instructor. Employees are required are required to pass the course before they progress beyond probation.

The course, held whenever there are five (5) or more new employees in the department, covers all aspects of materials management and key facets of support service programs:

1. Purchasing
2. Inventory control
3. Supply distribution
4. Infection control
5. Safety
6. Patient supply charges
7. Sterilization
8. Material processing
9. Quality control
10. Customer service
11. Effective communications
12. Body mechanics
13. Computer system use (as applicable to job responsibilities)

On successful completion of the course, participants receive a certificate that denotes satisfactory participation.

Affected Departments

Reviewed _____

Subject	Effective Date 1-90	Latest Revision & Date
EVALUATION OF EMPLOYEE PERFORMANCE		

An employee's performance is evaluated periodically, based on scope of responsibilities and measurable accountabilities:

1. After the first 90 days of employment, to determine whether the employee should be advanced beyond probationary status

2. After the first six months of employment

3. After the first full year of employment

4. Annually thereafter

5. Periodically, as determined by the manager

The evaluation does not necessarily mean the employee will receive a wage increase. If the evaluation is unsatisfactory, an increase would not be granted.

In the case of poor performance, the employee will be counseled and trained further. If the poor performance continues, the employee may be placed on probation or, eventually, dismissed.

Affected Departments

Reviewed _____

<u>MATERIALS MANAGEMENT EMPLOYEE RECORD</u>

NAME _____   HIRE DATE _____

POSITION _____   RATE OF PAY _____

                                         (DATE) _____

                                         _____

Date(s)	Subject: Inservice Evaluation Counseling	Presented By	Comments/Results

Subject	Effective Date	Latest Revision & Date
INFECTION CONTROL	1-90	

Materials management follows infection control principles in accordance with guidelines set by state and federal agencies and the Joint Commission on Accreditation of Health Care Organizations. The institution's environmental services committee and infection control surveillance officer assist in establishing acceptable standards, procedures, and environment.

The materials management infection control program includes:

1. Strict, physical separation between clean and soiled areas.

2. Air handling systems that provide an effective deterrent to airborne transportation of bacteria. All soiled areas have <u>negative air pressure</u> so that air does <u>not</u> flow out of these areas. All clean areas have <u>positive air pressure</u> so that soiled air does not flow into them.

3. Separate material flows. The cart lift transports clean supply carts at one time and soiled items/carts at a separate time.

4. Isolated pneumatic tube system for internal, enclosed transport of soiled linen and trash. Linen and trash are transported automatically to their pickup and disposal points.

5. Thorough cleaning of all areas on a scheduled, regular basis.

6. Utilization of quality control system for in-house sterilization (sterilizer monitoring) that includes chemical, biological, and mechanical monitoring of equipment; lot numbering; and product-recall capabilities.

7. Routine cultures taken on samples of commercially purchased sterile supplies.

8. Written procedures for external/internal product recall.

9. Strict enforcement of personal hygiene principles among employees, especially frequent hand-washing.

10. Strict enforcement of employee dress code in soiled and sterile processing areas. This includes gloves, masks, etc., when dealing with potentially infectious materials.

11. Strict traffic control in soiled and clean areas.

12. Central processing of all reusable utensils, surgical instruments, and patient care equipment. Processing is accomplished in the most economical and effective manner, using sophisticated equipment and up-to-date techniques.

13. Preventive maintenance on all processing equipment to ensure proper decontamination of used items.

14. Written isolation processing procedures.

Affected Departments

Reviewed _____

Subject	Effective Date 1-90	Latest Revision & Date
DEPARTMENT CLEANING		

The department will be cleaned by housekeeping personnel according to the schedule below:

Area	Type—Frequency—Time
Decontamination	Wash walls—as needed—evenings Wet mop floors—daily—evenings Wash ceilings—semiannually—evenings
Bathroom/locker	Wet mop floors—daily—evenings Wash fixtures—daily—evenings Wash ceilings/walls—semiannually—evenings
Preparation and packaging	Wet mop floors—daily—evenings Wash ceilings/walls—semiannually—evenings
Linen pack room	Wet mop floors—daily—evenings Wash ceilings/walls—semiannually—evenings
Sterile stores	Wet mop floors—daily—evenings Wash ceilings/walls—semiannually—evenings Dust shelves—daily—evenings
Processed stores	Wet mop floors—daily—evenings Wash ceilings/walls—semiannually—evenings Dust shelves—daily—evenings
Dispatch office	Wet mop floors—daily—evenings General office cleaning—daily—days
Equipment storage	Wet mop floors—daily—evenings Wash ceilings/walls—semiannually—evenings
Print shop	General office cleaning—daily—evenings
Bulk stores	Wet mop floors—daily—days Wash walls—annually—days Dust shelves—daily—days
Mail room	General office cleaning—daily—days
Stores bathroom	Wet mop floors—daily—days Wash fixtures—daily—days

Affected Departments

Reviewed _____

Subject	Effective	Latest
DEPARTMENT CLEANING (cont.)	Date 1-90	Revision & Date

Receiving dock
Wet mop floors—daily—days
Wash walls—annually—days

Trash room
Wet mop floors—daily—days
Wash compactor (exterior)—daily—days

Linen room
Wet mop floors—daily—days
Wash walls—annually—days

Purchasing
General office cleaning—daily—evenings

Archives
Wet mop floors—daily—days
Wash walls—annually—days

Soiled hold room (4)
Wet mop floors—daily—days
Wash walls—as needed—days
Wash fixtures—daily—days
(Includes trash/linen tube chutes)

Clean hold room (4)
Wet mop floors—daily—days
Wash walls—semiannually—days
Wash fixtures—daily—days

Cart lifts (3)
Wash—daily—days

Nurservers (196)
Wash weekly—as needed (20 per day per floor)

Materials management personnel will be responsible for periodic dusting and straightening of shelves. Spills will be wiped up immediately by materials management personnel if housekeeping personnel are unavailable.

Materials management will clean all equipment items according to the following schedule:

1. Terminal sterilizers—daily
2. Washer/sterilizers—daily
3. Dish machine—daily (after each meal)
4. Cart washer—weekly
5. Sonic cleaner—daily
6. Work stations and countertops—daily

Any requests for special cleaning will be made through the manager to housekeeping personnel.

Affected Departments

Reviewed _____

Subject		Effective Date 1-90	Latest Revision & Date
REPORTS			

The following reports are prepared by materials management on a regular basis.

1. Overtime log

Record of overtime incurred and approved. Submitted by each manager as requested.

2. Lost supply charges report

Summary/total of all lost patient supply charges by each patient care area (nursing floor). Prepared monthly and submitted to the director of nursing, the vice-president of finance, and the president for review.

3. Linen poundage report

Verification of invoices submitted by the commercial laundry against the hospital's records. Submitted monthly to accounting as authorization to pay the invoice.

4. Linen usage report

Summary/total of linen used (in pounds) by each department (cost center). Submitted monthly for review by administration, affected department heads, and managers.

5. Quality assurance report

Evaluation of the department's performance. Prepared by each manager monthly and submitted to the director and, possibly, to the president for review and analysis.

6. Materials management annual report

Summary of major accomplishments, improvements, or cost savings achieved by the department during the past calendar year. Submitted to the president for review.

7. Purchasing vendor analysis

Evaluation of vendor's performance based on quality and quantity factors. Prepared annually by purchasing for review with the vendors.

8. Purchasing annual report

Summary of activity and analysis of volume, costs, etc. Prepared annually by purchasing for the vice-president of finance and the president.

9. Print shop report

Summary/total of all copies made monthly and then annually by the copiers and printing press.

Affected Departments

Reviewed _____

Subject	Effective Date 1-90	Latest Revision & Date
CONFLICT OF INTEREST		

All members of the materials management staff are expected to support and abide by the institution's policies on conflict of interest.

These include:

1. Refusal of all gifts and gratuities from vendors, patients, and any other parties. Allowance will be made for business meals. The institution will periodically (every other time) pay for the entire meal or at least the meal of institutional staff.

2. Pursuit of, participation in, or ownership of (direct and indirect [spouse or family member], partial or total) any business venture or activity that:

   a. The institution might do business with

   b. Would create or be suspected of creating a distraction from the full attention to and time availability for the position and responsibilities for which the employee has been hired and is compensated

   c. Would bring about financial gain such that it could become the employee's primary interest or vocation

3. Decisions that are not solely in the institution's best interest.

4. All products, software, programs, etc., that are developed while in the employ of the institution, for the benefit or use of the institution; these shall remain the sole property of the institution unless expressly agreed to, in writing, by both parties, before any such effort is initiated.

Affected Departments

Reviewed _____

Subject	Effective Date 1-90	Latest Revision & Date
CONFIDENTIALITY		

Per institutional policy, all information and data about patients, staff, operations, plans, performance, methods, assets, and so on are considered completely confidential and will not be discussed or disclosed, in whole or in part to any outside parties or unauthorized staff until, if ever, that information is available in the public domain.

Professional judgment and discretion should always be used.

Affected Departments

Reviewed _____

Subject	Effective Date 1-90	Latest Revision & Date
PERFORMANCE MEASUREMENT AND MANAGEMENT		

Materials management has established measurable and manageable indicators and standards used to evaluate departmental, functional, and individual performance.

The following facets are measured monthly:

1. Service
2. Costs
3. Control
4. Productivity

A multifaceted report is prepared for review and action by the following:

1. Senior management/administration
2. Key customers (surgery, nursing, laboratory)
3. Materials management staff and management team

Performance is evaluated against the standards and compared with the previous month, quarter, and fiscal year.

Affected Departments

Reviewed _____

Page 1 of 1

PERIOD ENDING _____

PURCHASING
PERFORMANCE ANALYSIS

		PERIOD			Y-T-D	
MEASURE	**INDICATOR**	**PLAN**	**ACTUAL**	**VARIANCE**	**PLAN**	**ACTUAL**	**VARIANCE**

Volume of activity
- Dollars spent
- P.O./lines
- Bids/quotations
- Requisitions/lines
- Sales interviews
- Phone calls
- Shipments/lines

Labor/productivity
- Hours paid
  - —Regular
  - —Premium
- Hours worked
  - —Regular
  - —Premium
- Lines/hour

Costs
- P.O.
- Line
- Patient day
- Function
- Total
- Percent of hospital

Quality/performance
- Days to process order
- Order error
- Price index
- Late deliveries
- Invoice discrepancies
- Price-protected contracts
- Products evaluated/standardized

PERIOD ENDING _____

INVENTORY MANAGEMENT
PERFORMANCE ANALYSIS

	PERIOD			Y-T-D		
	PLAN	ACTUAL	VARIANCE	PLAN	ACTUAL	VARIANCE

MEASURE

Volume of activity

Labor/productivity

Costs

Quality/performance

INDICATOR

Dollar investment
Transactions
—Receipts
—Issues
—Additions
—Deletions
Line items

Hours paid
—Regular
—Premium
Hours worked
—Regular
—Premium
Transactions/hour

Carrying costs
Obsolescence
Transaction
Patient day
Total
Percent of hospital

Dollars per bed
Turns rate
Stock fill rate (percent)
Shelf-to-file errors
File-to-g/l errors
Stock-outs

PERIOD ENDING _____

STORAGE AND DISTRIBUTION
PERFORMANCE ANALYSIS

MEASURE	INDICATOR	PERIOD			Y-T-D		
		PLAN	ACTUAL	VARIANCE	PLAN	ACTUAL	VARIANCE
Volume of activity	Receipts/lines/pieces						
	Shipments/lines						
	Orders/lines						
	Carts/lines						
	"Emergency" orders/lines						
	Credits/returns						
	Dollars issued						
	Space (square feet)						
Labor/productivity	Hours paid						
	—Regular						
	—Premium						
	Hours worked						
	—Regular						
	—Premium						
	Lines/hour						
	Pieces/hour						
	Carts/hour						
	Deliveries/hour						
Costs	Line						
	Patient day (classification)						
	Function						
	Total						
	Percent of hospital						
Quality/performance	Order error rate						
	Late deliveries						
	"Emergency" orders						
	Square feet per bed						
	Damaged/destroyed items						

PERIOD ENDING _____

SUPPLY CHARGES
PERFORMANCE ANALYSIS

	PERIOD			Y-T-D		
	PLAN	ACTUAL	VARIANCE	PLAN	ACTUAL	VARIANCE

MEASURE	INDICATOR
Volume of activity	Transactions
	Charges—in and outpatient
	Credits—in and outpatient
	Additions
	Deletions
	Total revenue ($)
	Inpatient
	Outpatient
	Total credits ($)
	Inpatient
	Outpatient
	Lost charges
	Total charges lost ($)
	Net revenue ($)
	Inpatient
	Outpatient
Costs	Total costs
	Per charge
	Per patient day
	Lost charges/patient day
Quality/performance	Error rate
	Lost charges
	Revenue/charge
	Gross margin (percent)
	Revenue/patient day
	Revenue/ER/OR procedure
	Percent of hospital revenue

PERIOD ENDING _____

MATERIAL PROCESSING
PERFORMANCE ANALYSIS

	PERIOD			Y-T-D		
	PLAN	ACTUAL	VARIANCE	PLAN	ACTUAL	VARIANCE

MEASURE	INDICATOR
Volume of activity	Cycles/loads
	—Sonic
	—Washer/sterilizer
	—Sterilizer
	—Cart wash
	Sets/packs wrapped
	Sets/packs assembled
	Orders/lines
	Case carts
	Equipment
Labor/productivity	Hours paid
	—Regular
	—Premium
	Hours worked
	—Regular
	—Premium
	Cycles/hour
	Lines/hour
	Carts/hour
	Packs/hour
Costs	Item
	Patient day
	Surgical procedure (by type)
	Function
	Total
	Percent of hospital
Quality/performance	Set/pack errors
	Order errors
	Cart errors
	Positive cultures
	Equipment malfunctions

61

PERIOD ENDING _____

LAUNDRY/LINEN SERVICE
PERFORMANCE ANALYSIS

		PERIOD			Y-T-D	
	PLAN	ACTUAL	VARIANCE	PLAN	ACTUAL	VARIANCE

MEASURE

Volume of activity

INDICATOR

Pounds processed (all types)
Orders/lines
Carts/lines
Repaired pieces
ID marked pieces
Packs made

Labor/productivity

Hours paid
—Regular
—Premium
Hours worked
—Regular
—Premium
Pounds/hour
Lines/hour
Pieces/hour

Costs

Replacement
Pound
ER/OR procedure
Patient day (classification)
Surgical procedure
Line
Function
Total
Percent of hospital

Quality/performance

Late deliveries
Order errors
"Emergency" orders
Rewash/stains—pounds
Replacement percent
Pounds per patient day
Pounds per surgical procedure

SECTION II

PURCHASING
SECTION II

Subject	Effective Date	Latest Revision & Date
PURCHASING MISSION AND SCOPE OF SERVICES	1-90	

The purchasing office is responsible for procuring all the supplies, equipment, and services required for operations and patient care in a timely and cost-effective manner. This includes inventory supplies, noninventory (direct) departmental supplies, capital and minor equipment, parts and accessories, and services.

The purchasing office is solely authorized to commit institutional funds for any purchase. This committal is accomplished by issuing a purchase order (see sample), signed by the purchasing manager, or a designee (buyer).

Orders are not considered binding, nor will respective invoices be paid, without a corresponding purchase order and receiving report.

The purchasing office provides product and price information to in-house departments as requested or as it becomes available. All contracts with vendors must be made through purchasing. This applies to sales representatives who call for appointments with various departments.

Purchasing also negotiates contracts in conjunction with the departments that require service for equipment.

Affected Departments

Reviewed _____

PURCHASE ORDER

PURCHASE ORDER NO.

TO:

SHIP TO

BILL TO:

DATE
VENDOR NO

TAX EXEMPTION

THE HOSPITAL IS EXEMPT FROM STATE SALES TAX. THE TAX EXEMPT NUMBER IS:

☐ IF X'ED, THIS IS A CONFIRMING ORDER – DO NOT DUPLICATE –

PURCHASE ORDER INSTRUCTIONS

1 SPECIFIED TERMS AND CONDITIONS APPEAR ON THE REVERSE SIDE HEREOF. ANY DEVIATIONS MUST BE AGREED UPON IN WRITING BEFORE THIS CONTRACT IS BINDING

2 PURCHASE ORDER NUMBER MUST APPEAR ON ALL INVOICES, PACKING SLIPS AND ANY OTHER CORRESPONDENCE REGARDING THIS ORDER

3 DELIVERIES SHOULD BE MADE TO THE HOSPITAL RECEIVING DOCK ONLY. RECEIVING HOURS ARE 7:30-4:00pm. MONDAY THROUGH FRIDAY. SATURDAY AND SUNDAY DELIVERIES WILL BE MADE TO THE DOCK AND HANDLED BY THE DISPATCH OFFICE

4 SHIPPING TERMS ARE F O B HOSPITAL. IF THESE CONDITIONS ARE NOT ACCEPTABLE. SHIPMENTS MUST BE MADE ON A PREPAID AND ADD TO INVOICE BASIS AND MUST BE AGREED UPON IN WRITING BY THE BUYER

5 INVOICES SHOULD BE SENT TO THE ABOVE STATED "BILL TO" ADDRESS

6 NON-DISCRIMINATION - THE NON-DISCRIMINATION CLAUSE CONTAINED IN SECTION 202 OF THE EXECUTIVE ORDER 11246 AS AMENDED BY THE EXECUTIVE ORDER 11375 RELATIVE TO EQUAL EMPLOYMENT OPPORTUNITY FOR ALL PERSONS WITHOUT REGARD TO RACE, COLOR, RELIGION, SEX OR NATIONAL ORIGIN AND REGULATIONS PRESCRIBED BY THE SECRETARY OF LABOR ARE INCORPORATED HEREIN

F O B - HOSPITAL	DELIVERY DATE		SHIP VIA	INVOICE TERMS			SHIP ON OR BEFORE		FOR HOSPITAL USE ONLY		
ITEM NO	QUANTITY	PURCH/SHIP UNIT	DESCRIPTION		UNIT PRICE	EXTENDED PRICE	HOSP ITEM # COST CENTER #	QUANTITY	DISPENSING UNIT	DISPENSING UNIT COST	
1											
2											
3											
4			SAMPLE								
5											
6											
7											
8											
9											
10											
11											
12											
13											
14											

DIRECTOR OF PURCHASING

VENDOR COPY

Subject	Effective Date	Latest Revision & Date
PURCHASE REQUISITION AUTHORIZATION	1-90	

In an effort to control requisitions for stock and special-order supplies, each department will complete and return an authorization form (see below). The list of people authorized to sign requisitions must be up-to-date. All requisitions signed by unauthorized persons will be returned to the issuing department.

From: _____   _____
                (Department)   (Date)

TO: Purchasing Office

RE: Personnel Authorized to Requisition/Order Supplies

Honor requisitions for <u>stock</u> supplies signed by:

_____   _____
Type name   (Signature)   Type name   (Signature)

_____   _____
Type name   (Signature)   Type name   (Signature)

NOTE: All requisitions for nonstock direct purchase items must be reviewed and approved by:

_____
(Signature) Manager or department head

Affected Departments

Reviewed _____

Subject	Effective Date	Latest Revision & Date
AUTHORIZATION FOR PURCHASING	1-90	

The purchase of supplies, equipment, and services for institutional use is the responsibility of the purchasing office and staff. Pharmaceuticals and food products may be ordered by the pharmacy and dietary departments, respectively, with previous approval of the president and board of directors.

Purchases are confirmed and binding only on completion of a signed purchase order. An invoice will be paid only if it can be matched with a purchase order that has been authorized and processed.

Purchases for supplies and equipment are generally authorized in advance as a part of the fiscal year's budget. Nonbudgeted or emergency items are evaluated for approval by administration as they occur.

The purchasing manager [or, in his or her absence, the appropriate designee(s)] is authorized by the president and board of directors to commit institutional funds for goods and services purchased. The purchasing functions (product research, negotiation, closing, etc.) are coordinated or conducted solely by the purchasing manager or staff, except for the following:

1. Contracts for consultants' services, auditors, temporary staff, etc.
2. Donations
3. Construction; as designated by the president (see Procedure #2.37)
4. Employment contracts
5. "Specialty" items (i.e., major x-ray equipment/systems, major laboratory equipment/systems, computers, etc.); as designated by the president, other members of the senior management staff may conduct the research and investigation after a purchase order has been set aside. The purchasing manager will lead the final negotiations and closing.

Administration and department heads may request purchasing to proceed with purchases within the following limits of authority and with appropriate signatures:

1. Department heads:

   a. Routine, budgeted supplies
   b. Routine, budgeted parts, service/repairs, and equipment

Affected Departments

Reviewed _____

Subject	Effective Date	Latest Revision & Date
AUTHORIZATION FOR PURCHASING (cont.)	1-90	

2. Administration representatives and vice-president of finance:

   a. Nonbudgeted items for their respective departments
   b. Emergency items for their respective departments
   c. Nonroutine or major equipment
   d. Major repairs or service
   e. Major supply contracts (semiannually or annually) over $500

3. Vice-president of finance and president:

   a. Approved, budgeted, capital expenditures up to $100,000
   b. Emergency expenditures up to $30,000

4. Board of directors:

   a. Capital expenditures over $100,000

The above limits are reviewed annually and adjusted for inflation, as necessary.

Affected Departments

Reviewed _____

Subject	Effective Date	Latest Revision & Date
PURCHASE OF STOCK (INVENTORY) ITEMS	1-90	

The purchasing office obtains the information on what stock items to order and when, from three sources:

1. The <u>computer action summary report</u>—a report listing all stock items that require attention (below minimum, above maximum, etc.). The items are listed in numerical order, by vendor, so that purchase orders can be prepared from the list.

2. The <u>computer going-to-order report</u>—a report listing items that will probably reach reorder point within the next week. The items can be prepared from the list.

3. The <u>computer whole file item-status report</u>—a report listing all stock items and their status.

The purchasing buyer reviews the reports and uses the following stock buying procedures:

1. Monday/Thursday:

   a. Review computer action summary for items that must be ordered.
   b. Verify in the open order file or on the open order report that they have <u>not</u> been ordered.
   c. Verify order placed by drawing a yellow line through it on the computer action summary report. Also write in the purchase order number assigned on the computer action summary.
   d. Produce a purchase order through the computer system.
   e. Phone in order, present to sales representative, or electronically transmit it to the vendor.

2. Daily:

   a. Review computer whole file item-status and computer zero/last-on-shelf reports for any zero items.
   b. Verify if item is on order. If it is not, order it. If it is, expedite it.

3. Wednesday/Friday:

   a. Review computer whole file and computer zero reports for items that need action.
   b. Make out computer load and changes for any corrections or revisions required.
   c. Expedite open file/open order reports.
   d. Follow up on any problems.

Affected Departments

Reviewed _____

Subject	Effective Date	Latest Revision & Date
PURCHASE OF STOCK (INVENTORY) ITEMS (cont.)	1-90	

The following information is required for each purchase order:

1. Purchase order number
2. Vendor name
3. Vendor address
4. Vendor code number
5. Item/stock number
6. Item description
7. Item dispensing unit
8. Item unit cost
9. Item extended cost
10. Total line items ordered
11. Total units ordered (quantity)

NOTE: Only two (2) purchase orders may be placed for any one item at a time. The computer will not accept any more purchase orders until one is received or canceled.

Any price changes noted at the time the order is placed should be noted in the file and on the face of the purchase order copies in the appropriate space.

Copies of the purchase order are disseminated in the following order:

1. White confirmation copy to the vendor
2. Goldenrod copy to purchasing's open file
3. Yellow copies (3) to receiving
4. Pink copy to accounting
5. Green copy for data entry by the inventory control clerk

The inventory control clerk will obtain verification that orders have been placed by referring to the computer system's transactions report. The other daily and weekly reports used to place the purchase order are retained for 30 days as a source of reference so that purchasing knows which items have been ordered.

Once purchase orders have been entered, they will be summarized on the open orders report when they have gone beyond their expected delivery date. This facilitates follow-up and expediting procedures.

Affected Departments

Reviewed _____

Subject	Effective Date	Latest Revision & Date
INVENTORY CONTROL	1-90	

The purchasing office has a major role in inventory control.

The purchasing office orders inventory supplies as they are needed (when reorder point is reached). The status of inventory items is reported to purchasing either through the computer system or written communications from storeroom personnel. Purchasing's responsibility is to respond to that information and obtain the goods as quickly and economically as possible.

In addition, purchasing has major input into the inventory control system for establishing reorder points and reorder quantities based on delivery lead times, quantity discount and contract purchases, promotional sales, and institutional cash-flow conditions.

Purchasing is responsible for authorizing or correcting price or quantity discrepancies on all vendors' invoices.

Affected Departments

Reviewed _____

Subject	Effective Date 1-90	Latest Revision & Date
PURCHASE OF NONSTOCK (DIRECT) SUPPLIES		

The healthcare institution requires authorization and documentation to purchase supplies and equipment used for in-house operations, both for budgeted and nonbudgeted (emergency) purchases.

Department heads (and/or their designees) are authorized to approve purchases for routine items on their own signature. (See Procedure #2.2.)

Requests for nonroutine or high-value items or equipment must be authorized and signed by the department head, the administrative representative for the department, and the controller/vice-president of finance, before presenting them to purchasing. This includes the purchase of any capital or major equipment. (See Procedure #2.8.)

The requesting department will obtain a nonstock request for purchasing services form (see sample) and provide the following information:

1. Date submitted
2. Date required by item
3. Quantity required
4. Complete description of item(s) required, including manufacturer, vendor, catalog number, model number, etc.
5. Any acceptable substitutes
6. Department name, cost center number, and expense account number
7. Brochures when possible

NOTE: A separate form must be filled out for unrelated items and for each different vendor.

Authorization signatures must be obtained before submitting the form to purchasing. Orders without the correct signatures will be returned to the requesting department before the order is placed.

When the form is completely filled out and signed, the department should:

1. Retain the yellow copy for its own records and follow-up
2. Present the white and pink copies to purchasing

Affected Departments

Reviewed _____

Page 1 of 2

Procedure #2.6

NONSTOCK REQUEST FOR PURCHASING SERVICES*

PURCHASING DEPT.

SELECT ONE

- ORDER
- PRODUCT INFORMATION
- RETURN
- RENT
- BORROW

*THIS IS NOT AN ORDER - FOR INTERNAL USE ONLY.

ITEM NO.	QUANTITY	UNIT	PRODUCT NO.	DETAILED DESCRIPTION OF PRODUCT-SERVICE	VENDOR #1	VENDOR #2	VENDOR #3
					▶	▶	▶
1							
2							
3							
4							
5							
6							
7							
8							
9							
10							
11							

DATE SUBMITTED _____

DATE REQUIRED _____

REQUESTED BY _____

DEPARTMENT NAME _____

APPROVED BY _____   DATE _____

DEPT NO _____

PURCHASE ORDER NO _____

☐ ORDER IS CONFIRMING

EXPECTED DELIVERY DATE

ORDERED BY _____

75

Subject PURCHASE OF NONSTOCK (DIRECT) SUPPLIES (cont.)	Effective Date 1-90	Latest Revision & Date

The purchasing buyer uses the following nonstock buying procedures:

1. Verify authorizing signatures, department name, cost center number, etc.; if not complete, return to department
2. On receipt of the request, stamp date "received in purchasing" on the face of the form
3. If order is more than $500, obtain at least two (preferably three) competitive prices
4. Until order is placed (maximum of three working days from the date received in purchasing), place request in the nonstock hold bin
5. When the order is placed, note the expected delivery date on the purchase order and the request
6. Tear apart the purchase order and distribute copies; place the purchase order in the open order tub file
7. Place the request for purchasing services (white copy) in the nonstock request file, by department
8. Return the request for purchasing services (pink copy) to the requesting department, with the purchase order number, vendor, expected delivery date, and price information included
9. Follow up or expedite when the due date is reached or when requested by the user department

When the item is received, the receiving clerk should inspect the item against the packing slip and purchase order.

The item is presented to the ordering department for final inspection, and the authorizing signature is placed on the receiving report, which is then forwarded to purchasing. Purchasing notes on its control copy (goldenrod) that the item has been received and forwards the receiving report to accounting.

The accounting department matches the receiving report with the invoice from the vendor before any payment is made. Any discrepancies are brought to the attention of purchasing for investigation before payment.

Affected Departments

Reviewed _____

Subject	Effective Date	Latest Revision & Date
TRAVELING CARD PURCHASES	1-90	

The traveling (requisition) card is used to make repeat, nonstock purchases of items that are used regularly but are not stored in the storeroom. It is not used for "one time" purchases.

The traveling card contains purchase and usage information for a given item. (See sample.)

A department wishing to use the traveling card to request a purchase fills out the card with:

1. Vendor name
2. Item name
3. Item catalog or model number
4. Item cost (per unit)
5. Quantity requested
6. Department name
7. Cost center number and budget account number
8. Date requested
9. Date required
10. Signature

The card is forwarded to purchasing, where the date received is marked on the card. If the card is properly completed, purchasing prepares a purchase order within three working days.

Any information obtained from the vendor (delivery date, price change, etc.) is noted on the card when the order is placed, along with the date ordered and the purchase order number. The card is returned to the requesting department.

Follow-up or expediting is done when the due date is reached or when the user department requests it.

When the order is received, the department notes this in the space provided on the card. When it is time to reorder the item, the cycle repeats.

Affected Departments

Reviewed _____

Page 1 of 1

TRAVELING (REQUISITION) CARD

DEPT._____ DEPT. No.:_____

NOMENCLATURE:_____

SPECIFICATIONS:_____

_____

UNIT OF ISSUE:_____

MIN._____ MAX._____

CHARGEABLE ☐   NON-CHARGEABLE ☐

ALTERNATE VENDORS	VENDOR NAME	VENDOR No.	VENDOR ADDRESS		VENDOR STOCK No.	PACKAGE QTY.	LATEST COST	CONTRACT
			FOR PURCHASING DEPARTMENT USE ONLY					

DATE REQUESTED	QUANTITY REQUESTED	REQUESTED BY	DATE ORDERED	QUANTITY ORDERED	P.O. NUMBER	LATEST COST	VENDOR	DATE RECEIVED	QUANTITY RECEIVED

DATE REQUESTED	QUANTITY REQUESTED	REQUESTED BY	DATE ORDERED	QUANTITY ORDERED	P.O. NUMBER	LATEST COST	VENDOR	DATE RECEIVED	QUANTITY RECEIVED

Subject	Effective Date	Latest Revision & Date
PURCHASES, CAPITAL EXPENDITURES (EQUIPMENT, RENOVATION, SUPPLIES)	1-90	

Capital items are anything with a unit cost of $300 or more or a useful life of three (3) years or more.

Purchases of capital items (furniture, equipment, service or renovation, etc.) are budgeted whenever possible. These require justification in writing, completion of a request for purchasing services form, and authorization by the department's vice-president, the vice-president of finance, and the president.

The purchasing office is authorized and responsible for managing the process used for capital expenditures (equipment, supplies, services).

Budgets for capital expenditures are prepared annually, for a three-year period, per American Hospital Association (AHA) guidelines. The capital expenditure committee is a subcommittee of the finance committee of the healthcare facility's board. It includes the following members:

1. President
2. Vice-president of operations
3. Vice-president of finance
4. Director of materials management
5. Vice-president of medical affairs/chief of staff
6. Vice-president of nursing/patient care services
7. Vice-president of clinical services

Any expenditures exceeding $100,000 must be reviewed and approved by the finance committee of the board.

The capital budgeting process begins in June each year. Completion is scheduled for October so that activities for the upcoming fiscal year can be initiated appropriately. The process is as follows:

1. Departments develop complete lists of expected capital equipment needs and submit them to administration and materials management.

2. Director of materials management meets with department heads to discuss their capital equipment needs.

3. Director of materials management helps department head determine general specifications for equipment. Vendor information may be required in this process. Director of materials management should compile vendor product information.

4. Director of materials management obtains estimated prices for capital equipment meeting the general specifications.

Affected Departments

Reviewed _____

Page 1 of 2

Subject	Effective Date	Latest Revision & Date
PURCHASES, CAPITAL EXPENDITURES (EQUIPMENT, RENOVATION, SUPPLIES)	1-90	

5. Director of materials management should assist department head in completing a capital equipment request form. (Exhibit A)

6. Administration, with the director of materials management, reviews all of the capital equipment requests and selects the equipment to be approved. An approved capital equipment list is developed including the quarter during which each item will be purchased.

7. Director of materials management presents the approved capital equipment list at a department head meeting and requests input regarding potential problems, or possibilities for coordination or schedule changes.

8. At least two months prior to the quarter during which each capital equipment item will be purchased, the director of materials management meets with the department head to plan the purchase process. (Exhibit B)

9. Detailed equipment specifications are developed, expanding on the general specifications developed previously.

10. A request for proposal is prepared listing the specifications and terms of purchase. The request should be reviewed by the director of plant operations to determine if the space planned for the equipment will be appropriate: for example, utilities available, sufficient space available for maintenance access, etc.

11. Director of materials management sends the request for proposal to potential vendors.

12. Director of materials management and department head review responses. Director of materials management negotiates with vendors, arranges for evaluations, if necessary, and selects and notifies winning vendor.

13. Director of materials management arranges for delivery and installation of equipment.

14. Director of materials management meets with department head to determine if equipment is operating correctly and to review the purchase process.

Affected Departments

Reviewed _____

EXHIBIT A
CAPITAL EQUIPMENT REQUEST FORM

CAPITAL EQUIPMENT REQUEST

Department _____   Request #_____
                                                         (Assigned by purchasing)
Date _____

Submitted by_____   Approved by _____
                   Department head

Fill out one form for each single piece of equipment costing over $ _____ or for each group of equipment costing over $ _____ . Complete each section. Use additional pages if necessary to expand on any information requested.

I.   Item description _____

     Approximate purchase cost_____

     Lease cost, if available _____

II. Describe what the equipment does, how it will be used in your department, and the benefits that it will provide. If the equipment will improve worker productivity, reduce operating expense, or improve quality, give specific projections of the impact of the equipment on your operating expenses.

     _____
     _____
     _____
     _____
     _____
     _____
     _____
     _____
     _____

III. Does this replace an existing piece of equipment?   Yes_____ No _____ If yes, describe the existing piece of equipment and explain why it needs replacement. Include, where appropriate, maintenance history, changes in technology or standard practice, regulatory agency citations.

     _____
     _____
     _____
     _____

IV. How frequently will the item be used, how many times per day, per month, or per year, and how long will it be used each time it is used?

     _____
     _____

EXHIBIT A
CAPITAL EQUIPMENT REQUEST FORM (cont.)

V. What will be the impact of the equipment on the institution's marketability? Will it bring new patients or physicians and/or prevent loss of patients or physicians? _____ _____ _____

VI. Are there special requirements for the equipment? Address issues such as humidity, temperature, ventilation, electricity, plumbing, special gases. _____ _____ _____

VII. What would be the consequence on your department if this piece of equipment is not purchased this year?_____ _____ _____

VIII. Provide any other information that is relevant to a decision regarding acquisition of this piece of equipment. _____ _____ _____ _____

IX. Financial Summary
Part 1:   Projected annual revenue from the equipment _____

Detailed operating expenses:

Annual cost of supplies to operate the equipment   _____

Annual cost of maintenance for the equipment (after the warranty expires), include parts, labor, service contract, etc.   _____

Annual cost of labor to operate the equipment   _____

Annual cost of utilities to operate the equipment   _____

Expected life of the equipment   _____

Annual depreciation   _____

Total annual costs   _____

Net profit from the equipment: revenue less expenses   _____

Will the equipment replace an existing piece of equipment?   Yes_____   No_____   If yes, complete Part 2.

EXHIBIT A
CAPITAL EQUIPMENT REQUEST FORM (cont.)

Part 2:   Is the existing equipment fully depreciated?   Yes_____   No_____

If no, the remaining depreciation is _____ and the annual depreciation

is _____ .

The actual revenue from the existing equipment is _____ .

Detailed operating expenses:

Annual cost of supplies to operate the equipment   _____

Annual cost of maintenance for the equipment (after
the warranty expires), include parts, labor, service
contract, etc.   _____

Annual cost of labor to operate the equipment   _____

Annual cost of utilities to operate the equipment   _____

Expected life of the equipment   _____

Annual depreciation   _____

Total annual costs   _____

Net profit from the equipment: revenue less expenses   _____

EXHIBIT B
CHECKLIST TO ADDRESS
IN CAPITAL EQUIPMENT PURCHASE PROCESS

Positions Involved in Review	Check When Done	Function in Equipment Purchase Process
Administration	☐	Approves purchase and specifies timing of purchase
Department director	☐	Initiates request
	☐	Develops specifications with assistance of the director of materials management
	☐	Completes Capital Equipment Request Form with assistance of the director of materials management
	☐	Reviews bids, evaluates proposed equipment
	☐	Approves those vendors' proposals that are acceptable
Physicians who would use the equipment	☐	Provide clinical input on development of specifications
	☐	Test equipment and provide input on the clinical evaluation of the equipment
Director of plant operations	☐	Reviews equipment specifications, and proposals if necessary, to determine if the equipment will operate satisfactorily in the space intended; checks utilities available, space for maintenance, capacity of air handling, etc.
	☐	Reviews equipment to make sure it meets safety requirements
Other department heads	☐	Review equipment requests to determine if it may be possible to coordinate two or more purchases or if any conflicting goals and objectives exist for different equipment purchases

Features/terms to address:

☐ Payment of freight

☐ Cost of installation

☐ Cost of maintenance contracts

☐ Arrangements for servicing, both during normal hours and after hours

☐ Contract for purchase of supplies and/or replacement parts to be used with equipment

☐ Warranty arrangements

☐ Liability arrangements

☐ Inservicing arrangements

☐ Arrangements for testing of equipment

☐ Contract for additional or replacement equipment

☐ Contract for equipment upgrades

Subject	Effective Date	Latest Revision & Date
ASSET/PROPERTY CONTROL	1-90	

The institution maintains records on all assets that it owns/purchases for control and managment analysis purposes.

An asset is described as any property item the hospital owns that is:

1. Worth more than $300
2. Not a fixed item (i.e. built-in cabinet, equipment, etc.)
3. Not an expendable supply
4. Not leased or rented
5. Useful for three (3) years or longer

Control is achieved by:

1. Placing a property tag on each item
2. Recording the item on a record form
3. Keeping a file for each department listing all the items for which it is responsible

The tag, placed in an inconspicuous place on the item, visually identifies the item as institutional property.

The tags are nonremovable and numbered so that each item can be identified. (See sample.)

Each item purchased/owned is recorded on the asset/property record that includes a complete description, the number assigned, the date purchased, dollar value, and the department responsible for it. (See sample.)

Each department is responsible for all asset items purchased by or assigned to it. Any permanent movement from the departmnet, maintenance required or performed, disposal, or trade-in must be reported so that records may be maintained accurately.

The records are used by accounting for budget, insurance, and depreciation purposes; by purchasing to determine when such items are available; and by maintenance for repair and replacement decisions. Copies of the reocrds are maintained in each of the above areas. Each area is responsible for updating its own records. (Maintenance will keep files only on items that require maintenance or parts.)

Affected Departments

Reviewed _____

Subject	Effective Date 1-90	Latest Revision & Date
ASSET/PROPERTY CONTROL (cont.)		

When the purchasing office orders assets, it will prepare the asset/property records, obtain the necessary number of property tags, and forward the purchase order, tags, and asset/property records to receiving.

Receiving will hold documents in the open file until the items arrive.

When the items arrive, receiving will attach the tags in an inconspicuous but consistent place, complete the asset/property record, forward copies to purchasing, accounting, and maintenance (as necessary), and deliver the items to the user department.

Purchasing, accouting, and maintenance will file the asset/property record in the file by department responsible (not by item type). Any changes of status on the item are recorded and include:

1. Permanent move to another department
2. Maintenance or other repairs
3. Trade-in
4. Scrap
5. Sale

Departments requesting maintenance, disposition, repairs, new parts, or accessories should refer to the property number of the item so all records can be accurately updated.

Periodic inventories will be taken by all in-house departments to update and verify asset/property records.

Disposition of assets through trade-in or sale is based on the value of the item as shown on the asset/property record.

Affected Departments

Reviewed _____

PROPERTY TAG

Property of
HOSPITAL NAME
#15124

Property of
HOSPITAL NAME
#15125

ASSET/PROPERTY RECORD

CODE	PROPERTY TAG #

ITEM DESCRIPTION (include color, size, fabric)

MODEL #	SERIAL #	MANUFACTURER
DEPARTMENT NAME		COST CENTER #
LOCATION (BUILDING)	FLOOR	ROOM #

TRANSFERRED TO: LOCATION (Department #/Room #)	DATE
TRANSFERRED TO: LOCATION	DATE
TRANSFERRED TO: LOCATION	DATE

COMMENTS

_____

_____

_____

_____

PURCHASED FROM VENDOR	COST (Dollars)
PURCHASE ORDER #	DATE

EXPECTED LIFE	DEPRECIATION	
DISPOSITION DATE	AMOUNT	METHOD

Subject	Effective Date	Latest Revision & Date
DISPOSITION OF ASSETS/PROPERTY AND OTHER OBSOLETE ITEMS	1-90	

The disposal of excess equipment and other materials will be handled by purchasing.

Departments will notify purchasing of anything to be offered for sale, including silver recovered from x-ray film, scrap paper, etc.

Purchasing will decide, after consulting whatever sources are necessary, whether it will be more financially advantageous to sell a piece of equipment or to scrap it. This includes determining the cost of a new piece of similar equipment, obtaining a professional appraisal, and setting a realistic selling price for the equipment.

In buying updated equipment of the same type, purchasing will ask if the old equipment can be traded-in. If the equipment is not honored as a trade-in, it will then be listed on a bulletin to be distributed to a group of other healthcare institutions, industrial users, or any others likely to have a use for the item, including in-house employees.

All offers will be received by purchasing and reviewed by the purchasing manager and the vice-president of finance before being accepted.

The sale will be accomplished by presenting an outgoing report form to the business office with the item's description and selling price posted on the form. The item will be paid for and the buyer given a PAID receipt for the item (or the report is marked PAID). Purchasing will file the top copy in the retired assets/property file and give a copy to the buyer. The asset/property record will note that the item has been sold, to whom, and for how much. In the case of materials, the department's revenue account will be credited for the amount of the sale.

With major purchases, an invoice billing may be prepared and issued to the buyer and other terms may be arranged. All this will be documented on the outgoing report form.

The goods will then be released to the buyer.

Affected Departments

Reviewed _____

Page 1 of 1

Subject	Effective Date	Latest Revision & Date
PURCHASE OF ELECTRICAL EQUIPMENT	1-90	

Unless otherwise authorized by the institution, the following requirements apply to all purchases of electrical/electronic equipment and systems:

1. Electrical:

   a. Units will be capable of operating with line fluctuations of 115V ± 10 percent, 208V ± 10 percent, 60HZ ± 1HZ.
   b. Units will be capable of operating for extended periods in a 20 to 80 percent relative-humidity environment.
   c. Leakage current for patient-related equipment will be less than 10 µamps under normal operating conditions.
   d. Equipment for 115V operations will have three-prong, "U"-bar grounded plugs.
   e. Equipment will be specified with regard to line interference or any line loading during its normal operation.

2. Documentation:

   The supplier will provide:

   a. Two copies of an operating and service manual
   b. Schematics, wiring diagrams, logic and/or flow diagrams for the entire system
   c. A theory of operation, either found in one of the manuals or published separately
   d. Commercial vendor manuals for institutional use, where applicable

3. Warranty:

   The supplier will warrant or guarantee the equipment for one (1) year, unless indicated otherwise. Any exceptions will be noted on the purchase order or contract.

4. Proprietorship:

   The supplier will note all areas of proprietorship and outline a service agreement that will avoid hardship for the institution in case of equipment malfunction.

   In lieu of institutional specifications, all equipment will comply with the National Electrical Code, be UL listed, and meet OSHA regulations.

Affected Departments

Reviewed _____

Page 1 of 1

Subject	Effective Date 1-90	Latest Revision & Date
PURCHASE OF DIETARY PRODUCTS		

Purchasing is responsible for the purchase of all institutional supplies and equipment.

Food-service supply contracts are negotiated and approved jointly by purchasing and food service. Blanket or standing purchase orders are established where possible. In the case of daily or other frequent order needs (fresh foods), food service will release deliveries against previously negotiated (through purchasing) orders.

All nonfood purchases, such as equipment, paper supplies, chemicals, etc., are ordered through and by purchasing.

Food-service purchase orders and receiving reports are processed in the same manner as all other orders.

Affected Departments

Reviewed _____

Page 1 of 1

Subject	Effective Date 1-90	Latest Revision & Date
PURCHASE OF PHARMACY MEDICATIONS AND DRUGS		

Purchasing is responsible for the purchase of all institutional supplies and equipment.

The pharmacy orders drugs and other pharmaceuticals directly from suppliers selected through previous negotiation. Contracts with the suppliers were completed jointly by purchasing and the pharmacy.

The chief pharmacist is authorized to order only drug items. Other items required for the pharmacy must be obtained through purchasing.

Affected Departments

Reviewed _____

Subject	Effective Date	Latest Revision & Date
PURCHASE OF EMERGENCY ITEMS	1-90	

Purchasing is responsible for the purchase of all institutional supplies and equipment.

During normal business hours, 7A.M. to 5P.M., Monday through Friday, the following will be done:

1. Need for the emergency item will be verified by the department requesting it, and purchasing will learn exactly when the item is needed and how long the quantity will last.

2. The usual procedure for placing an order will be followed, except:

   a. Direct contact must be made with a party who can and will respond to the order (sales representative, customer service, sales manager, etc.). Do not give up until contact is made!
   b. The emergency status of the order must be explained, and it must be verified that the party realizes the exact nature of the situation.
   c. After the order has been confirmed, the requesting party will be advised in writing of all information regarding the item(s) [i.e., when and how the item(s) will arrive]. Do not give up until contact is made!
   d. Dispatch must be advised if the goods will arrive after receiving hours.

3. If unable to obtain items from a vendor, other healthcare institutions should be called, starting with the closest ones first. Once a source is found, transportation of the item(s) will be arranged, and the requesting party will be advised. Do not give up until contact is made!

During nonbusiness hours (evenings and weekends), emergency supplies and equipment will be obtained thus:

1. The area supervisor will contact the dispatch office to see if the supply item is available there. The exact item, quantity, use, time of need, and name of the patient must be provided.

2. If it is available in materials management, the item will be sent to the requesting department.

3. If the item is unavailable, the dispatcher (24 hours a day, 7 days a week) will contact surgery, emergency, and other in-house departments that store large quantities of supplies. If it is still not available, the dispatcher will contact local area healthcare institutions and local vendor representatives to try to locate the needed item(s).

4. If the item is located, the dispatcher will arrange for transportation via a hospital employee, taxicab, or bonded messenger service.

5. If the item is still unavailable or unlocated, the materials management manager on call will be contacted by the dispatcher, and, if necessary, the purchasing manager will be called.

After obtaining the item(s), all the pertinent information regarding the search for and acquisition of the item(s) must be recorded. This information is prepared by the person handling the situation and forwarded to purchasing when it reopens for business. This information will be used to prepare a purchase order and a nonstock request for purchasing services form as soon as possible.

The requesting department is responsible for coordinating follow-up with purchasing.

Affected Departments

Reviewed _____

Page 1 of 1

Subject		Effective Date 1-90	Latest Revision & Date
PURCHASE ORDER EXPEDITING			

The purchasing office maintains an open purchase order file for all open, incomplete orders. This file is alphabetical by vendor, numerical by purchase order number, and chronological.

Every week, the open purchase order file will be reviewed by the purchasing staff. All orders that are overdue will be pulled for follow-up.

Follow-up on an open purchase order requires:

1. Reviewing open order report for accuracy and acting on any items listed as past due

2. Reviewing open order file for any orders past due

3. Organizing purchase orders that need expediting by vendor

4. Calling vendor: sales representative, customer service personnel, sales manager, president of the company

5. Attempting to obtain the items immediately, or, if a long delay will occur, canceling the order and replacing that vendor with another source that can deliver faster (if available)

6. Making notes on the purchase order (goldenrod copy), including date, person contacted, nature of the delay, expected date of delivery, etc., and initialing the entries

7. Refiling the purchase orders in the open file

8. Advising the requesting party of the results in writing

Any order more than three (3) months old will be pulled from the open file and investigated for potential cancellation. If a delivery date cannot be agreed on or the problem(s) solved, a cancellation notice may be given to the vendor, after discussion with the requesting department.

Any reorder must be initiated by the requesting department.

Affected Departments

Reviewed _____

Page 1 of 1

Subject	Effective Date 1-90	Latest Revision & Date
PURCHASES/PETTY CASH		

The purchasing office is responsible for purchasing all institutional supplies and equipment.

A purchase order (contract) is prepared for every item purchased. The subsequent receiving report serves as the voucher by which accounting is authorized to pay the invoice for the respective item.

Because of the administrative cost of preparing and processing a seven-part purchase order, some small-dollar-value items (up to $20) may be purchased from a petty cash fund.

Department heads and supervisors authorized to make a purchase for in-house use without a purchase order will advise the purchasing office of their intent and discuss appropriate sources, will purchase the item, pay in cash, and obtain a paid receipt. This receipt is then presented to purchasing, where the employee obtains authorization for a cash reimbursement from the petty cash fund, located in the business office, cashier's window.

In all cases of cash purchases, the institution's tax-exempt number should be presented before the purchase so that taxes are not paid.

Affected Departments

Reviewed _____

Subject		Effective Date 1-90	Latest Revision & Date
PURCHASE ORDER PROCESSING			

All purchases of supplies and equipment, whether stock or nonstock, routine, special, or emergency, will be referenced at the time of order by a purchase order number.

Collect shipments on purchases will not be accepted unless previously arranged and noted on the purchase order. If premium routing is required, the healthcare facility will accept the billing.

Substitutions will not be allowed unless accepted by the department head or person using or ordering the goods.

Annually, a form letter will be sent to all suppliers and new vendors explaining that payment will not be made for shipments to the institution that are not authorized by a purchase order number and the signature of the purchasing manager or the director of materials management.

When a confirming copy of a purchase order is requested by a supplier, the purchase order will contain the statement "Confirming Order—Do Not Duplicate."

For electrical and electronic equipment, the general conditions for purchase of electrical equipment (see Procedure #2.11) will be included as part of the purchase order agreement, and a reference to that effect will be typed on the purchase order. Three copies of schematics will be required on these purchases.

An open purchase order file will be maintained in purchasing by the staff.

A closed, or completed, purchase order file will be maintained in the purchasing office and filed alphabetically by major suppliers, in purchase order number sequence for five (5) complete years. Only files for the last 18 months will be kept in the purchasing office. All purchase orders issued will be maintained in numerical sequence by the purchasing staff.

Any significant deviation from normal quantities or specifications must be checked thoroughly before placing an order.

Affected Departments

Reviewed _____

Subject	Effective	Latest
PURCHASE ORDER PROCESSING (cont.)	Date 1-90	Revision & Date

The purchase order (see sample) will be typed or printed on the computer system. It will include:

1. Complete vendor name and address
2. Special shipping instructions
3. Date
4. Terms
5. Quantity ordered
6. Institutional storeroom code number for all stock items
7. Complete description of each item
8. Unit price
9. Total price
10. Department head ordering the item
11. Name of department
12. Signature of purchasing manager

Orders for equipment will contain instructions regarding delivery, warranty, special conditions that may apply, any appropriate vendor quotation number, and a request for three copies of schematics on all electrical or electronic items.

When purchasing has been unable to determine a firm price, an estimated cost will be entered, followed by "EST." Expected or required delivery dates also are noted on the purchase order when possible.

Purchasing will distribute copies as follows:

1. The white copy of the purchase order will be mailed to a vendor only when the vendor requests it, or if the order is for capital equipment costing $100 or more. When not used as such, this copy of the purchase order is destroyed.
2. The goldenrod copy is retained for the open order file.
3. The pink copy is sent to accounting.
4. The three (3) yellow copies are sent to receiving.
5. The green copy is retained in the numerical sequence file, after it has been keypunched by data processing.

After receipt of goods, purchasing will:

1. Attach the receiving report (see sample) to the goldenrod copy; attach all packing slips and freight bills, if available, and forward the yellow copy of the receiving report to the accounting department. If the order is not complete, the second and third yellow copies of the purchase order will be retained by receiving for future partial shipments. If after the third partial shipment is received, the order is not complete, a subsequent receiving report will be made out and the third yellow copy retained by receiving until the final partial shipment is received. When the final partial shipment is received, the third yellow copy will be sent to accounting. Posting to the purchase record files will be made from the goldenrod copy, which is retained in purchasing.

Affected Departments

Reviewed _____

Subject	Effective Date	Latest Revision & Date
PURCHASE ORDER PROCESSING (cont.)	1-90	

2. When the order is complete, all packing slips, freight bills, etc., are stapled to the goldenrod copy and filed in the closed purchase order file, which is retained in purchasing.

Purchase orders are phoned to vendors or transmitted on the computer system. Copies of the purchase order are mailed to the vendor only for capital expenditures, for first-time ordering from a new vendor, and at the vendor's request.

For procedures on processing purchases through the computerized materials management information system (CMMIS), refer to the CMMIS manual.

Affected Departments

Reviewed _____

PURCHASE ORDER

TO:

SHIP TO:

BILL TO:

TAX EXEMPTION
THE HOSPITAL IS EXEMPT FROM STATE SALES TAX. THE TAX EXEMPT NUMBER IS:

DATE

VENDOR NO.

☐ IF X'ED, THIS IS A CONFIRMING ORDER
– DO NOT DUPLICATE –

F.O.B. – HOSPITAL

DELIVERY DATE

SHIP VIA

INVOICE TERMS

SHIP ON OR BEFORE

FOR HOSPITAL USE ONLY

ITEM NO.	QUANTITY	PURCH/SHIP UNIT	DESCRIPTION	UNIT PRICE	EXTENDED PRICE	HOSP. ITEM # COST. CENTER #	QUANTITY	DISPENSING UNIT	DISPENSING UNIT COST	QTY. REC'D	QTY. REC'D	QTY. REC'D
1												
2												
3												
4												
5												
6												
7												
8												
9												
10												
11												
12												
13												
14												

DATE | DATE | DATE

REC'D BY | REC'D BY | REC'D BY

DEPT. SKG. | DEPT. SKG. | DEPT. SKG.

INV.
TOTAL LINE
ITEMS ORDERED

INV.
TOTAL LINE
ITEMS REC'D

SAMPLE

DIRECTOR OF PURCHASING

ORDER COMPLETE ☐

PURCHASING DEPT. COPY

RECEIVING REPORT

SHIP TO

BILL TO:

TO:

PURCHASE ORDER NO.

DATE	DATE	DATE
REC'D BY	REC'D BY	REC'D BY
DEPT. SIG.	DEPT. SIG.	DEPT. SIG.
QTY. REC'D.	QTY. REC'D	QTY. REC'D

ORDER COMPLETE ☐

DATE

VENDOR NO.

TAX EXEMPTION

THE HOSPITAL IS EXEMPT FROM STATE SALES TAX. THE TAX EXEMPT NUMBER IS:

☐ IF X'ED, THIS IS A CONFIRMING ORDER
– DO NOT DUPLICATE –

SHIP ON OR BEFORE

FOR HOSPITAL USE ONLY

F.O.B. – HOSPITAL

DELIVERY DATE

SHIP VIA

INVOICE TERMS

ITEM NO	QUANTITY	PURCH/SHIP UNIT	DESCRIPTION	UNIT PRICE	EXTENDED PRICE	HOSP. ITEM # COST. CENTER #	QUANTITY	DISPENSING UNIT	DISPENSING UNIT COST
1									
2									
3									
4									
5									
6									
7									
8									
9									
10									
11									
12									
13									
14									

SAMPLE

INV. TOTAL LINE ITEMS ORDERED

INV. TOTAL LINE ITEMS REC'D

DIRECTOR OF PURCHASING

CONTROL COPY-RECEIVING

Subject	Effective Date	Latest Revision & Date
STANDING ORDERS	1-90	

The purchasing office negotiates annual contracts with vendors for quantities of supplies to obtain price protection and to lower the administrative costs of purchasing.

Standing (or contract) orders are set up for a maximum of one (1) year. Prices are guaranteed for that time, according to the terms of the purchase order. Quantities and delivery dates are determined by the purchasing manager, storeroom supervisor, and the department head involved (in the case of a nonstock direct purchase order). These terms are also included in the actual purchase order and are noted on the contract itself.

Once the purchase need has been determined, the department head must obtain authorization according to policy.

If the item is an inventory item, the purchasing manager negotiates the terms. The purchase order is then prepared.

If the terms of delivery require more than three (3) shipments during the life of the contract, as many copies of the receiving report as will be needed to document the extra receivings are made and attached to the original receiving reports and forwarded to receiving to await the first shipment. If ordered through the computer system, additional copies are not required.

The purchase order and the receiving reports are filed alphabetically by vendor and are reviewed approximately sixty (60) days before completion for possible renewal.

The receiving reports are processed exactly as any others, except when there will be more than three (3) partial shipments received. Receiving shipment numbers 4, 5, 6... etc., are noted by writing the appropriate number in the respective receiving report column. (See Equipment Receiving, Procedure #4.12.)

Affected Departments

Reviewed _____

Subject	Effective Date 1-90	Latest Revision & Date
INVOICE DISCREPANCIES/APPROVAL		

The purchasing office is solely authorized to commit institutional funds for supply and equipment items.

The purchase of these items is contracted with a vendor by a purchase order. The contract becomes binding when signed by the purchasing manager and received and accepted by the vendor.

Invoices are sent to the institution for goods ordered and received. Receipt is documented and verified by the receiving report, completed by the receiving clerk at the time goods are received.

The accounting department pays only those invoices that can be matched with a completed receiving report. Invoices are held until such proof of receipt is obtained.

If any discrepancy is noted on the invoice (price, quantity, etc.), the accounting department will not pay the invoice without consulting purchasing for verification and correction of the discrepancy.

Purchasing will research the problem by contacting receiving or other in-house personnel and the vendor for proof of delivery or explanation of any price discrepancies. Purchasing will document the explanation, authorize acceptance and payment, or reject the invoice, then forward the signed documentation to accounting.

Affected Departments
_____

Reviewed _____

Page 1 of 1

Subject	Effective Date	Latest Revision & Date
PURCHASES FOR NONPATIENTS	1-90	

The institution follows ethical and regulatory guidelines regarding the resale of products purchased under the Robinson-Patman Act. The institution allows purchases of medical supplies for employees on a limited basis; that is, only those items unobtainable from commercial/retail sources.

Purchasing will provide information on sources of supply as a benefit to employees and the medical staff.

Outpatients and ready-to-be-discharged patients may purchase medical supply items if the items are unavailable from other sources.

Once a sale is established as above, purchases are made by:

1. Reporting to the business office/cashier and identifying the item(s) to be purchased

2. Obtaining from the purchasing office the selling price (institution's cost) as listed in the price master or stock catalog

3. Reporting to the business office with a completed outgoing report form that lists the price and paying for the item(s) with cash only

4. Obtaining from the business office a paid receipt that notes the item(s), quantity, price, purchaser's name, and date

5. Picking up the item(s) at the cashier's office

Affected Departments

Reviewed _____

Page 1 of 1

Subject		Effective Date 1-90	Latest Revision & Date
	RETURNS OF PURCHASED ITEMS		

The purchasing office coordinates the shipment of the following:

1. Defective items being returned to the vendor
2. Incorrect shipments being returned in exchange for correct items
3. Over or double shipments being returned to the vendor
4. Shipments to charities, or other donations officially sent by the institution
5. Miscellaneous shipments that are official institutional business

A department wishing to return or ship supplies or equipment is required to provide the following information on a nonstock request for purchasing services form (see sample) to purchasing:

1. Department requesting shipment
2. Items to be shipped
3. Quantity to be shipped
4. Reason for shipment
5. Destination (vendor name and address)
6. Date purchased
7. Approximate value (for insurance purposes)

This information, forwarded to purchasing, is documented on an outgoing report. (See sample.)

Purchasing forwards a copy of the outgoing report to the accounting department to notify it of the intent to return items so that an invoice is not paid. The report also alerts accounting to watch for the vendor's incoming credit. The accounting department also will arrange to credit the department's budget account for the value of the return or credit.

The purchasing office will notify the requesting department when the above has been completed so that it may arrange for the receiving personnel to pick up and prepare the items for shipment. If the items can be hand-carried, the requesting department is expected to take them to the receiving area.

Purchasing will prepare any shipping labels or insurance forms required for the appropriate number of packages and forward them to the receiving area for the goods. A copy of the outgoing report form is sent to receiving to be used as a packing slip.

The receiving personnel prepare a packing slip/bill of lading for the shipment. They contact the appropriate common or private carrier to arrange for pickup and transport.

The receiving personnel record all data pertinent to that shipment on the shipping log.

After the goods are shipped, any subsequent problems with the shipment, credit to be received, etc., are handled by purchasing.

Affected Departments

Reviewed _____

NONSTOCK REQUEST FOR PURCHASING SERVICES

SELECT ONE	
	ORDER
	PRODUCT INFORMATION
	RETURN
	RENT
	BORROW

*THIS IS NOT AN ORDER - FOR INTERNAL USE ONLY.

ITEM NO.	QUANTITY	UNIT	PRODUCT NO.	DETAILED DESCRIPTION OF PRODUCT-SERVICE	VENDOR #1	VENDOR #2	VENDOR #3
					▶	▶	▶
1							
2							
3							
4							
5							
6							
7							
8							
9							
10							
11							

DATE SUBMITTED _____

DEPARTMENT NAME _____

DEPT NO _____

EXPECTED DELIVERY DATE _____

DATE REQUIRED _____

APPROVED BY _____ DATE _____

PURCHASE ORDER NO _____

ORDERED BY _____

REQUESTED BY _____

☐ ORDER IS CONFIRMING

105

OUTGOING REPORT

IMPORTANT!

THE REFERENCE NUMBER LISTED BELOW MUST APPEAR ON ALL PACKAGES, SHIPPING PAPERS, INVOICES, CREDITS AND OTHER CORRESPONDENCE

REFERENCE NUMBER

TO:

DATE:

THE REASON FOR SHIPMENT OF THE ITEMS LISTED IS:

- [ ] RETURN FOR EXCHANGE
- [ ] RETURN FOR CREDIT
- [ ] SENT FOR REPAIR
- [ ] RETURN TO LENDER/RENTER
- [ ] LOANED*
- [ ] INCORRECT ITEM RECEIVED
- [ ] SALES*
- [ ] OTHER*

* HOSPITAL is absolved of any liability resulting from the use of any items lent or sold

SHIPPED VIA: CARRIER

/ PREPAID OR COLLECT

- [ ] DELIVERED
- [ ] PICK-UP
- [ ] OTHER

ITEM NUMBER	QUANTITY	UNIT	PRODUCT NO.	DESCRIPTION	UNIT PRICE	AMOUNT
1						
2						
3						
4						
5						
6						
7						
8						
9						
10						
11						
12						
13						
14						

TOTAL NUMBER OF PIECES

RECEIVED BY   OUTGOING DATE

DRIVER

SHIPPING CLERK   RETURN DATE

Subject	Effective Date	Latest Revision & Date
PRODUCT RECALLS	1-90	

The purchasing office coordinates the recall of all suspect or defective goods immediately on receipt of notification from the manufacturer/vendor involved. If notification is received by mail, the mail clerk will make the appropriate number of copies for distribution to those listed.

When such notification is received, purchasing will immediately contact dispatch, storeroom, pharmacy, and nursing service to obtain assistance with the recall.

At this time, copies will be made of the notification and forwarded to administration and all users or suspected users of the item(s).

Personnel from these areas will personally visit user departments, inspect the area for the items, and remove any suspect items found. These will be taken to the holding area in receiving and put in quarantine.

Also at this time, purchasing will contact the representative of that company to determine disposition of the affected goods and obtain credit or acceptable replacements as soon as possible.

Purchasing will notify all affected departments about the availability of replacements.

Affected Departments

Reviewed _____

Subject	Effective Date	Latest Revision & Date
PRODUCT SUBSTITUTIONS	1-90	

During product shortages, transportation delays, etc., purchasing may be unable to procure the exact product requested by in-house departments.

If a product is unavailable, purchasing reserves the right and has the responsibility to obtain a worthy, effective substitute.

The purchasing office maintains an up-to-date master list of all supply items used in the institution. It is cross-referenced by item, vendor, and user department(s). For each item listed, users are required to provide at least one (1) acceptable substitute that purchasing may obtain, without contacting the users for further authorization in shortage or delay situations.

In cases of direct-purchase items for which substitutes are not known by purchasing, the buyer will ask for possible substitute products/sources and offer alternatives whenever possible. When feasible, purchasing will try to obtain items from other user departments or area healthcare facilities.

User departments will be notified of substitutions as soon as possible after the items have been ordered. This will be done either by purchasing or storeroom personnel.

Affected Departments

Reviewed _____

Page 1 of 1

Subject		Effective Date 1-90	Latest Revision & Date
PRODUCT INFORMATION REQUESTS			

In-house departments may require information on products for use in budget preparation or purchasing decisions.

Purchasing is responsible for obtaining and disseminating product information, both as requested and as a general operating procedure.

When requesting specific product information, the department manager should obtain and prepare a request for product information form. (See sample.)

This form is forwarded to purchasing, which obtains the necessary/requested information. The completed form is returned to the requesting department and a copy is kept on file in purchasing.

Any follow-up should be initiated by the concerned department.

Affected Departments

Reviewed _____

REQUEST FOR PRODUCT INFORMATION

TO: PURCHASING OFFICE

FROM_____   _____
(DEPARTMENT NAME)   (COST CENTER #)

REQUESTED BY _____   DATE _____
(DEPARTMENT HEAD/MANAGER)

INFORMATION   ☐ PRICE QUOTATION   ☐ BROCHURE(S)
REQUESTED   ☐ SAMPLE(S)   ☐ SEE REPRESENTATIVE(S)
                   ☐ Other _____

PRODUCT NAME_____

USE _____

_____

MANUFACTURER(S)   1. _____   3. _____
VENDOR(S)
                   2. _____   4. _____

PROVIDE THE FOLLOWING WHEN AVAILABLE:

       MODEL #_____   CATALOG #_____

       SIZE _____   ACCESSORIES_____

       *ELECTRICAL   _____
        REQUIREMENTS_____

       COLOR_____   OTHER_____

       *Requires review/approval by maintenance prior to evaluation/purchase
_____

DATE REQUESTED	VENDOR	PRICE	DATE RECEIVED
_____	_____	_____	_____
_____	_____	_____	_____
_____	_____	_____	_____
_____	_____	_____	_____

COMMENTS _____

_____

SIGNED_____   DATE _____
(PURCHASING MANAGER)

Subject	Effective Date	Latest Revision & Date
PRODUCT EVALUATION/STANDARDIZATION	1-90	

The product evaluation/standardization program has the following objectives:

1. Identify and select products and equipment used throughout the institution that provide acceptable levels of quality at the lowest possible cost, through a value analysis process
2. Bring about standardization that will reduce procurement and inventory carrying costs

The product evaluation/standardization committee has the responsibility and authority to make product selection and use decisions after a thorough analysis. Appeals of decisions may be taken to the management team.

The committee members include representatives from:

1. Materials management
2. Nursing management
3. Medical staff
4. Surgery
5. Finance
6. Support services
7. Clinical services

Members are appointed by the president and, usually, vice-presidents. The chairperson is appointed annually; the position is rotated among all members.

Serving the committee as consultants, on an as-needed basis, are:

1. Infection control
2. Biomedical engineering
3. Nursing education

Working with the committee are the following subcommittees:

1. Surgery
2. Diagnostic services
3. Nursing/medical staff

These subcommittees are responsible for:

1. Conducting evaluations
2. Recommending decisions to the committee
3. Completing follow-up research on committee decisions and actions

Affected Departments

Reviewed _____

Subject	Effective Date	Latest Revision & Date
PRODUCT EVALUATION/STANDARDIZATION (cont.)	1-90	

Subcommittee members are appointed by the committee chairperson. Each subcommittee will have no less than five (5) and no more than nine (9) members. The full committee meets monthly. The subcommittees meet as needed.

Vendor representatives are not allowed to make presentations at committee or subcommittee meetings. Interested members or parties will be expected to present items for consideration.

Communications of the committee and subcommittee include:

1. Publication of prior meeting minutes seven (7) working days before meetings
2. Publication and distribution of minutes to all in-house departments
3. Notification of decisions/actions to parties that request a review
4. Announcements of actions and accomplishments in the institution's newsletter
5. Follow-up surveys to users of selected products and equipment to validate decisions

Parties seeking evaluation of a product will obtain a request for product evaluation form (see sample) from purchasing. The form is completed and presented to any committee member (but preferably the chairperson) to be reviewed and placed on the next available agenda.

The committee and subcommittees will use the following forms (see samples):

1. Product evaluation form
2. Results report
3. Results survey

Affected Departments

Reviewed _____

REQUEST FOR PRODUCT EVALUATION

TO: PURCHASING MANAGER

FROM _____   SIGNED_____
                (DEPARTMENT)   (DEPARTMENT HEAD)

DATE _____

REASON FOR REQUEST

1. Product complaint

   Product name _____

   Product manufacturer _____

   Problem (please be specific) _____

   _____

   _____

   _____

   Solution suggestions

   _____ Replacement of item   _____ Re-Inservice

   Suggested replacement(s)/better product(s)

   Name _____   Manufacturer _____

   Name _____   Manufacturer _____

2. New product evaluation

   Product name _____

   Product manufacturer _____

   Product use _____

   _____

   Advantages _____

   _____

   _____

Date received by purchasing manager _____

Date scheduled for committee agenda _____

PRODUCT EVALUATION FORM

General data (purchasing and requesting department)

Item name _____   Manufacturer(s) _____

Catalog/model # _____   _____

Vendor(s) _____   _____

☐ Disposable   ☐ Reusable _____   Estimated usage _____

Basic use _____   Signature _____

_____   Date _____

Financial data (accounting department)

Unit cost _____   Labor costs _____ hours @ _____
                   (reprocessing)

Support supply cost(s)   Total $ _____ per unit of use

    Item/quantity _____   @ $ _____   Total $ _____

    _____ $ _____ $ _____

    _____ $ _____ $ _____

                   Total supply cost $ _____

☐ Patient charge $ _____   ☐ Nonpatient charge

Revenue analysis/pay-back period _____

_____

_____

                Signature _____

                Date _____

Storage/control data (materials management)

Shipping unit _____   Dispensing unit (for stock only) _____

☐ Replacing currently used item   ☐ New item   ☐ Stock item   ☐ Direct

☐ Single department use   Name of department _____

☐ Multidepartment use   Name of departments _____

_____

Initial order/evaluation quantity _____   Signature _____

PRODUCT EVALUATION FORM (cont.)

<u>Electrical/mechanical data</u> (engineering)

☐   Meets OSHA and UL requirements   Problems _____

☐   Compatible with current   _____
      institutional systems

Modifications necessary _____

_____

_____

Estimated cost of modifications $ _____

                                     Signature _____

                                     Date _____

<u>Product data</u>	Highly Acceptable	Acceptable	Not Acceptable	Rater's Signature
Patient safety				
Employee safety				
Packaging				
Handling				
Compatibility				
Space requirements				
Inservice required				
Disposability				

PRODUCT EVALUATION FORM (cont.)

Medical/technical
data

Highly Acceptable	Acceptable	Not Acceptable	Rater's Signature

Rater's comments _____

_____

_____

_____

_____

Rater's signature _____

<u>PRODUCT EVALUATION FORM (cont.)</u>

☐ Item rejected   ☐ Item approved

☐ Item approved for evaluation   ☐ Stock item—
                                            stock # assigned _____

    Evaluation period _____

                                         ☐ Direct purchase item

Evaluating department _____

       _____

Comments _____

_____

_____

_____

Date _____   _____
                                  (CHAIRPERSON, PRODUCT EVALUATION COMMITTEE)

PRODUCT EVALUATION COMMITTEE
RESULTS REPORT

TO _____
(REQUESTING DEPARTMENT)

FROM _____
(CHAIRPERSON, PRODUCT EVALUATION COMMITTEE)

DATE _____

PRODUCT _____ MANUFACTURER _____

RESULTS

_____ Approved for use   _____ Not approved   _____ Approved for trial only

COMMENTS_____

_____

_____

_____

_____

_____
(SIGNED)

PRODUCT EVALUATION COMMITTEE RESULTS SURVEY

TO: Staff member   Date _____

FROM: Product evaluation committee   New product name _____

Please complete this survey and return it to the purchasing office by the end of this week.

1. This product is: a. Better than expected   c. Unacceptable
   (circle one)   b. Adequate   d. Better than the one it replaced

2. If the product is better than expected, why? _____

_____

_____

3. If the product is unacceptable, why? _____

_____

_____

4. Was the inservice adequate?   Yes   No

5. Did you know about the arrival of the product before you were in a position to use it?

                                              Yes   No

6. Do you feel you need more time . . . (circle appropriate answer)

                    a. To evaluate the product properly?
                    b. To learn how to use the product properly?

7. Any other comment or items you would like to see the product evaluation committee look into?

_____

_____

_____

Subject	Effective Date	Latest Revision & Date
VENDOR RELATIONS/SALES AND SERVICE REPRESENTATIVES	1-90	

The following policy governs the activity of all sales and service representatives who do business with the healthcare institution:

1. All sales representatives wishing to contact in-house departments and personnel must do so through purchasing. Representatives are not to contact supervisors, department heads, or medical or nursing staff members directly. Requests for appointments and statements of reason for business must be made through purchasing.

2. Sales representatives include those individuals who market products to the institution. Service representatives are those who provide warranty or repair service for specialized equipment.

3. All sales and service representatives doing business with, or anticipating doing business with, the institution must enter and leave by the main entrance.

4. Sales representatives will not be allowed in the hospital after 4:30 p.m. unless prior arrangements have been made for such activities as product fairs/demonstrations or inservice programs.

5. Each representative will receive a copy of the purchasing policies regarding hospital relations and guidelines.

6. All representatives will report to purchasing (or to the information desk after hours), sign the register, and pick up a pass before proceeding to other departments.

7. All representatives must return their passes and sign out in the register before leaving the building.

Affected Departments

Reviewed _____

Subject	Effective Date	Latest Revision & Date
VENDOR CONTRACT NEGOTIATIONS	1-90	

The purchasing department is responsible for executing all institutional procurement contracts, including: service contracts, maintenance contracts, lease/rental agreements, etc.

The exceptions are employment and consulting contracts, which the president alone authorizes.

Departments involved with such contracts will prepare a request for purchasing services form and obtain the required authorized signatures before beginning any negotiations. The department(s) will then meet with purchasing to further discuss requirements.

The purchasing manager will conduct the negotiations. The administrative representative or the department head may be involved in the negotiation process when indicated. In most cases, negotiations will be handled by the purchasing manager alone.

Before contract expiration, the purchasing manager will pull the purchase order and contact the affected departments to discuss the contract and begin the renewal process.

Departments experiencing problems or other unusual conditions regarding contracts are encouraged to advise the purchasing manager so that notations, which may influence future transactions with that vendor, can be made for future reference.

Affected Departments

Reviewed _____

Subject	Effective Date 1-90	Latest Revision & Date
GIFTS TO HOSPITAL AND STAFF		

Employees will not accept gifts, entertainment, or favors (other than promotional or advertising items of nominal value) from potential or current suppliers, of more than $25 in value. The Code of Ethics should be consulted for more details.

If a company's normal practice is to bestow gifts of greater value, those gifts may be accepted and used as door prizes at the annual holiday party or for general use. Cash donations to the development fund are acceptable and preferred. The director of development should be contacted for details.

Any questions regarding the value or use of any such items will be resolved by either the director of materials management or the president.

Affected Departments

Reviewed _____

Subject	Effective Date	Latest Revision & Date
VENDOR EVALUATION	1-90	

The purchasing manager will conduct evaluations of all vendors with whom the institution deals on a regular basis.

This analysis will be discussed with the user departments and with the vendors.

This is done in an effort to improve relations between the institution and its vendors.

Vendors will be evaluated on the following:

1. Responsiveness to emergencies
2. Creativity (helping the institution improve quality and reduce costs)
3. Adherence to policies (appointments, invoice processing, etc.)
4. Back orders
5. Invoice discrepancies
6. Committed pricing
7. Price increases
8. Order errors
9. Delivery lead times
10. Product support
11. Product packaging

Affected Departments

Reviewed _____

Page 1 of 1

Subject		Effective Date 1-90	Latest Revision & Date
	GROUP PURCHASING		

The hospital participates in a group-purchasing organization's program to obtain vendor discounts on products, equipment, and services used for patient care and operations.

The purchasing department takes advantage of these agreements to obtain the best price and to avoid time-consuming bids on group-contract items.

In cases where the price, product, or service from a nongroup contract vendor is preferable to that offered by the group contract vendor, the institution may consider a purchase from the nongroup contract vendor. Before such a decision is reached, it is discussed by the purchasing manager, the director of materials management, the vice-president of finance, and the president. The advantages and disadvantages of such action are seriously considered.

The institution will honor any contracts to which it has committed, without deviation. If a nongroup contract vendor approaches the institution with an offer that is better than that offered by the group, the institution will advise the group and the vendor to obtain a more attractive offer through the group. Vendors not wishing to participate in the group will not be considered.

Affected Departments

Reviewed _____

Subject	Effective Date 1-90	Latest Revision & Date
LENDING/BORROWING SUPPLIES AND EQUIPMENT		

Purchasing has primary responsibility for all items lent to or borrowed from the healthcare institution. Purchasing will make all contacts to coordinate the transaction.

Purchasing should be contacted during business hours and given all the information needed to obtain the item borrowed or to coordinate the lending to another institution:

1. Item name (manufacturer)
2. Item quantity
3. Needed by (department/person)
4. Date/time needed
5. Length of time needed
6. Source/destination
7. Person to contact
8. Telephone number

Purchasing will record all the above data on an outgoing report form. This form will accompany the person picking up or delivering the item(s) borrowed or lent. The necessary signatures are obtained, and the report form is returned to purchasing with the green copy going to the department involved. The original is filed in the purchasing open file for supplies lent to or borrowed from the institution.

When purchasing is closed, the dispatch office should be asked for assistance. (See Procedure #2.14.)

All equipment, supplies, etc., will be lent to or borrowed only from other healthcare institutions, not individuals. As indicated, patients, physicians, and others will be referred to the institution's home-care organization.

Affected Departments

Reviewed _____

Subject	Effective Date 1-90	Latest Revision & Date
PRICE CHANGE NOTIFICATION		

Purchasing will notify departments when a price change occurs. The notification form includes:

1. Name of vendor
2. Item or service
3. Date of change
4. Old cost/new cost
5. Packaging change if applicable
6. Date of notice or effective date

Change notifications will be sent to all user departments for evaluation of patient selling-price impact. Copies are sent to the accounting and data processing departments.

Affected Departments

Reviewed _____

Subject	Effective Date 1-90	Latest Revision & Date
PURCHASE ORDER CANCELLATIONS		

All purchase orders more than six (6) months old or more than sixty (60) days past the expected delivery date will be pulled from the open file for review. The need for the item will be discussed with the user department(s).

Purchasing will contact the vendors to discuss the pending cancellation. If the order cannot be filled within 10 days, it will be canceled. Purchasing will then send copies of the purchase order status change to accounting, receiving, and the requesting department (for nonstock direct-purchase items). (See sample.)

Any item canceled must be reordered by the initiating department if required.

Receiving and accounting will return their copies of the purchase order to purchasing. Purchasing will file them in a canceled purchase order file, to be maintained there for three (3) years.

Affected Departments

Reviewed _____

Page 1 of 1

PURCHASE ORDER STATUS CHANGE

TO:

FROM: PURCHASING OFFICE   DATE

VENDOR NAME _____

VENDOR ADDRESS _____

_____

CHANGE: ☐ PRICE   ☐ QUANTITY   ☐ SHIP DATE

             ☐ CANCELLATION   ☐ OTHER

COMMENTS _____

_____

_____

_____

_____

Please be advised that the above noted purchase order has been changed.

If the items have been canceled, they must be requested again before a new purchase order will be processed.

Thank you.

_____
(PURCHASING)

cc: Accounting department
    Receiving
    Requesting department

Subject	Effective Date 1-90	Latest Revision & Date
SERVICE CONTRACTS		

The purchasing manager is responsible for the negotiation of all contracts entered into by the institution.

For service or maintenance agreements, the user department will contact the purchasing manager when such a contract is requested. The purchasing manager will verify that a request for purchasing services form has been properly completed and authorized. In addition, the appropriateness of such a contract will be reviewed with engineering to determine if it can be provided more cost effectively from any other source, including the maintenance or biomedical engineering departments. Engineering will also review the terms and conditions proposed before execution of the contract.

When service work is performed, copies of all work tickets will be retained by the user departments and forwarded to purchasing for attachment to the contract, for future reference.

Department managers will send a copy of the work ticket(s) to accounts payable, with an authorized signature for payment.

Affected Departments

Reviewed _____

Page 1 of 1

Subject		Effective Date 1-90	Latest Revision & Date
	FORMS MANAGEMENT		

Forms are classified as any printed material to which information is added.

There are two types of forms: stock and nonstock.

Stock forms are stored in inventory and used by several departments. They are ordered by the purchasing office. They are assigned an inventory number (seven digits for use on the computer inventory system) that is printed on the face of each form in the lower left corner. Departments wishing to use these forms order them from the storeroom on a stock requisition.

Nonstock forms are printed for a department's singular use. They may be obtained from a vendor or printed on a copy/duplicator machine. They are assigned an identification number that consists of the department's cost center number and a sequential number (e.g., purchasing's number is 651; nonstock purchasing forms are numbered 651.001, 651.002, etc.). This number is printed on the lower left corner of all forms, along with the date of the last printing.

Requests for new forms—stock

Departments requesting new stock forms that will affect many departments present the following to the chairperson of the forms review committee, when possible, 15 weeks before the form is needed (to allow adequate time for artwork, printing, etc.):

1. Department name, department number (cost center)
2. Name of form requested
3. Short description of form's use
4. List of all other user departments with their corresponding approval/authorization (signature and date)
5. Estimated quantity used annually/monthly
6. Sample or drawing of the form, number of copies required, etc.

This is submitted on a request for item additions to/deletions from/changes to inventory form.

After the forms review committee has reviewed the request, purchasing will obtain proofs for final approval by the users and the committee. When approved, the item will be ordered and added to inventory.

Affected Departments

Reviewed _____

Subject	Effective Date	Latest Revision & Date
FORMS MANAGEMENT (cont.)	1-90	

Printed forms used for official purposes must be reviewed and authorized by the forms review committee before being put into use.

The forms review committee is composed of the following members:

1. Medical records
2. Materials management
3. Nursing/inservice
4. Systems and information services
5. Print shop
6. Ad hoc members when items affect them

The committee, chaired by the director of materials management, meets monthly to review requests for additions, deletions, or changes to forms and authorizes materials management (purchasing and the print shop) to coordinate any of the above decisions.

The committee also reviews existing forms for standardization, improvement, or elimination. A forms manual that assists in design, development, and the management program is maintained.

A file also is maintained in the print shop that includes a sample of all forms (used, deleted, proposed) with all information relative to the form(s). The information includes:

1. Design specifications
2. Use/purpose
3. Usage volume
4. Source of purchase
5. Quantity stored (order quantity, reorder point, etc.)
6. Authorization

Forms will be reviewed with the following criteria:

1. Function—duplicate or similar to existing form
2. Size—standard $8^1/_2 \times 11$, $5^1/_2 \times 8^1/_2$, 4×6, etc.
3. Color of paper
4. Color of ink (generally black)
5. Number of copies—analysis of use/need of each
6. Data processing applications—layout, imprinting, zone, etc.
7. Double-side usage
8. Punched—compatible with charts, medical records, etc.
9. Cost—print in-house or through a commercial vendor
10. Usage—volume, various departments

Affected Departments

Reviewed _____

Subject	Effective Date	Latest Revision & Date
FORMS MANAGEMENT (cont.)	1-90	

The user departments will be notified when the new form arrives. They will order these forms from the storeroom on a stock requisition, after the "old" forms are used up.

All forms will be printed with the date designated and the institution's stock number on the lower left corner.

Requests for new forms—nonstock

Departments requesting/needing a new nonstock form will design a draft, assign the appropriate number, determine estimated usage, and submit this information to the forms review committee chairperson with a print shop order form.

The forms review committee will review the request for duplications, etc., and will authorize the print shop to complete the order after cataloging the form.

Any difficulties with the form/request will be worked out with the user department(s).

The print shop normally requires a minimum of one week to process the order.

The number assigned is the department's cost center, followed by a sequential three-digit number starting with .001, .002, up to .999. The department assigns its own number based on the other forms it is already using. The department(s) will be notified if the number assigned is a duplicate. Another number will then be assigned.

The print shop maintains a file that contains a master copy of each form and a list of all forms for each department. This is filed by department/cost center, numerically. The print shop adds new forms to the list. A copy is sent to the user department and the chairperson of the forms review committee.

Revision of stock (inventory) forms

Revision of forms stored in inventory and used by more than one department must be coordinated by the department initiating the change.

All the necessary information must be submitted along with signatures from the affected department(s) (see requests for new forms—stock) to the forms review committee at least 15 weeks before the change is required to take effect. The request for item additions to/deletions from/changes to inventory form should be completed. The committee will meet with the requesting department(s) to review the request and authorize any revision.

After the above is completed, purchasing will process the change in the same manner as a new form. Departments will be notified when the revised form is available.

Affected Departments

Reviewed _____

Subject	Effective Date	Latest Revision & Date
FORMS MANAGEMENT (cont.)	1-90	

The user departments will use up the "old" form before the revised one is released for use.

If the revised form must be used before the old ones are used up, the remaining forms will be <u>charged to the user departments</u>.

<u>Revision of nonstock forms</u>

Departments may revise their own departmental nonstock forms, as necessary.

A new/revised master should be submitted to the print shop with notification that the revision supersedes the old master. The revised date (month/year) should be placed on the lower left corner of the form near the form nonstock number.

The print shop will note the change in the forms manual and the date it was authorized.

<u>Deletion of stock (inventory) forms</u>

Departments wishing to delete forms that are obsolete may do so when necessary.

Materials management may contact user departments when inventory records indicate little or no usage of forms and request deletion.

In either instance, the deletion will be initiated on a request for item additions to/deletions from/changes to inventory form. All such requests are forwarded to/reviewed by the forms review committee, which notes the deletion in the files.

The user department(s) will be charged for all unused, deleted forms. They may use or dispose of them.

<u>Deletion of nonstock forms</u>

User departments may delete a nonstock form at any time by discontinuing its use. They will then send a notice to the print shop to delete the form and "retire" the form number.

The print shop will notify the forms review committee of the deletion and update the master file. The master of the deleted form is retained, and the date deleted is noted.

Affected Departments

Reviewed _____

Subject	Effective Date	Latest Revision & Date
PURCHASING CATALOGS	1-90	

The purchasing office maintains vendor catalogs for its own and other departments' use.

Departments and their personnel may use the catalogs during office hours in the purchasing office waiting room.

If the person wishes to use the catalog in another department, he or she will complete an "out card" with name, department, and date.

Subject		Effective Date	Latest Revision & Date
CONSTRUCTION PURCHASE ORDERS		1-90	

Supplies and equipment purchased as part of new construction, major renovation, etc., are obtained through the use of a construction purchase order form. (See sample.)

The president or senior vice-president will designate which items are to be purchased in this manner after all items are reviewed and approved.

A master list will be prepared and submitted to purchasing for preparation of the purchase order. (These purchase orders also may be prepared by administration or facilities planning, depending on the terms of the contract between the institution and the architect.)

The construction purchase order will contain exact specifications for the items below:

1. Quantity
2. Item description (size, color, model number, etc.)
3. Safety specifications: i.e., UL listed, flame retardant, etc.
4. Unit price
5. Total amount
6. Shipping terms
7. Expected delivery date
8. Installation terms
9. Warranty terms
10. Acknowledgment/invoice instructions

When completed, the purchase order is forwarded to the purchasing manager for his or her signature.

Copies are then distributed to:

1. President's office—goldenrod
2. Accounting—open file—yellow
3. Purchasing—control/open file—green
4. Receiving—control/open file—yellow and pink
5. Vendor for signature of acknowledgment—white, pink, green

NOTE: Files are maintained in alphabetical order by vendor.

Affected Departments

Reviewed _____

Page 1 of 2

Subject	Effective Date	Latest Revision & Date
CONSTRUCTION PURCHASE ORDERS (cont.)	1-90	

Acknowledgment copies are returned to accounting and maintained in the open file pending receipt of the goods and invoices.

Invoices are sent to accounting and held until a receiving report is processed.

Receiving indicates the arrival of the good(s) on the appropriate copies and forwards them to purchasing for posting on its open file copy. Purchasing then forwards that copy to accounting for invoice matchup and payment.

If additional copies are needed for receiving purposes, the extra acknowledgment copies will be obtained from accounting.

When the order has been completed, purchasing files its control copy in a construction purchase order closed file (alphabetical by vendor).

Problems with shipment, installation, acceptance, or invoice are handled by purchasing.

Affected Departments

Reviewed _____

CONSTRUCTION PURCHASE ORDER

DEPT. OF TAXATION EXEMPTION CERTIFICATE NO. ____

TO:

DELIVER TO:

MAIL FIVE-PART INVOICE TO:

P.O. #

P.O. DATE

SHIPPING INSTRUCTIONS:

MAIL ACKNOWLEDGMENT
COPY TO:

DELIVERY DATE
AT DESTINATION:

TERMS:

QUANTITY	CATALOG #	DESCRIPTION/INSTRUCTIONS	UNIT PRICE	AMOUNT

APPROVED

Construction manager
by _____ Date _____

Contractor
by _____ Date _____

Buyer
by _____ Date _____

ACCEPTED

Subject to other terms and
conditions on the reverse side

Seller
by _____
(Must be signed by corporate officer, partner,
or owner)

Date _____

Subject	Effective Date	Latest Revision & Date
SPECIALTY ITEM PURCHASES	1-90	

The president may delegate the lead responsibility to members of administration, other than the purchasing manager, to investigate the potential sources and specifications for a given piece or line of equipment when it is special (e.g., computers, x-ray, or laboratory equipment/systems). Purchasing will still be involved and will have the sole authority to consummate a contract/order with a vendor.

In this instance, a nonstock request for purchasing services form will be made out with the basic specifications and estimated costs. It is then signed by the president and forwarded to purchasing so that a purchase order is "set aside." The purchase order number will be written on the request form, which will be returned to administration. The pink copy of the request along with the purchase order will be placed in a hold file in the purchasing office.

After all information has been gathered, a time will be set for completing the order. The purchasing manager or director of materials management will meet with all parties involved to make sure all specifications and details have been completed to everyone's satisfaction.

The purchase order will be placed in the open file and processed like any other purchase order.

On receipt of the goods, the user department and the administrative representative will be contacted to verify satisfaction and sign the receiving report.

Any further problems will be handled by the administrative representative involved and the purchasing manager.

Affected Departments

Reviewed _____

Page 1 of 1

SECTION III

INVENTORY MANAGEMENT
SECTION III

Subject		Effective Date 1-90	Latest Revision & Date
INVENTORY MANAGEMENT PROGRAM			

Inventory is considered a valuable, manageable asset. Responsibility for managing inventory is delegated as follows:

1. "Official" storeroom inventory—materials management
2. Official pharmacy inventory—pharmacy
3. Official dietary inventory—dietary
4. Unofficial department inventory—each department

"Official" inventory is that inventory of consumable supplies that is considered as a current asset on the institution's balance sheet. It is counted and valued at least once each fiscal year.

"Unofficial" inventory is not carried on the balance sheet but represents a valuable asset. These consumable supply inventories are managed by department managers and may be counted and valued at fiscal year end (FYE) depending on their perceived value.

Inventories are maintained at their lowest possible level, balancing the need for maintaining continuity of supply to meet routine and peak demands with the interest in maintaining maximum cash flow.

Target annual inventory turns for each area are as follows:

1. Storeroom—15
2. Pharmacy—15
3. Dietary—30
4. Surgery—6
5. Critical care—35
6. Emergency—20
7. Radiology—25
8. Laboratory—20
9. Respiratory care—30

Managers will be held responsible for maintaining target levels and will be rated on inventory management as part of their annual performance evaluations.

For purposes of defining terms, stock items are those maintained in and by the storeroom. Nonstock items are maintained in and by the user departments. The mix of stock and nonstock items will be maintained at about a 60/40 ratio.

Affected Departments

Reviewed _____

Page 1 of 1

Subject	Effective Date	Latest Revision & Date
CRITERIA FOR OFFICIAL STOREROOM INVENTORY	1-90	

Because the healthcare facility is dealing with limited resources (dollars, space, etc.), criteria should be met in each request for new inventory items. If the criteria are not met, the item may not be placed into the storeroom inventory. The criteria to be used are:

1. Volume—the item must be withdrawn from inventory at least once a month. The inventory turnover rate for any stock item should be at least ten (10) per year.

2. Multidepartment use—an item may also be considered for stock when used by more than one area of the institution. The same brand will be used where possible.

3. Dollar value—when the value of the item(s) on hand exceeds $1,000, it may be beneficial to maintain the item(s) in the perpetual inventory instead of deducting a lump sum from a department's budget. This would properly allocate the budget and also provide historical data on that item.

4. Administrative cost—when the cost to maintain a supply item(s) in inventory (computer time, space, management time, data processing time, etc.) exceeds that of departmental cost, then the responsibility of maintaining the item should be turned over to the user department. (This would apply almost exclusively to single department users.) The reverse is true when the department's costs exceed those of keeping the item in stock.

5. Space—because space is limited to both the user departments and in the storeroom, the location with the most capacity should be the determinant. Therefore, when a department has enough room and the item is used solely by that department, the item should remain that department's responsibility.

6. Patient chargeability—all items that are directly patient chargeable will be set up in the inventory system.

Procedure Requests for Item Additions to/Deletions from/Changes to Inventory

Departments requesting additions to/deletions from/changes to storeroom inventory must fill out the request form (see sample) and submit it to purchasing for evaluation. Departments will be notified of the status of the request within ten (10) working days.

After all information and signatures are obtained on the form, items to be added to or deleted from inventory are prepared on a computer system inventory control complete load/change form. This form is prepared by the inventory control clerk, and the new stock number is assigned at that time (the check digit is included).

If the item is a patient chargeable supply from materials management, the selling price must be determined. (The finance department will determine the price formula.)

The stock or charge number (which must match) will be entered on the appropriate forms. The inventory control clerk will provide the information to the typist and see that the corrections are made/printed after the change, etc., has been processed by the computer.

Affected Departments

Reviewed _____

Subject	Effective Date	Latest Revision & Date
CRITERIA FOR OFFICIAL STOREROOM INVENTORY (cont.)	1-90	

New forms will be revised/printed when they reach reorder point, or at least quarterly, to incorporate all changes.

The departments will be notified of the changes, additions, and deletions by the storeroom. The storeroom will attach the item information (stock number, dispensing unit) to its next order.

The inventory control clerk will review the computer system's daily transactions report to verify that the item has been added or deleted properly.

Item changes such as description, dispensing unit, price, etc., are also completed on this request form. (See sample.)

Affected Departments

Reviewed _____

REQUEST FOR ITEM ADDITIONS TO/
DELETIONS FROM/CHANGES TO STOREROOM INVENTORY

TO: MATERIALS MANAGEMENT   DATE _____

REQUESTING
DEPARTMENT_____ REQUESTED BY _____

☐ ADDITION (NEW ITEM)   ☐ CHANGE (REPLACEMENT)   ☐ DELETION

ITEM
DESCRIPTION _____   STOCK #_____

USE/PURPOSE _____

_____

MANUFACTURER _____   VENDOR _____

CATALOG/MODEL # _____   PACKAGE/UNIT_____

COST _____   USAGE/MONTHLY_____

☐ PATIENT CHARGEABLE

☐ NONCHARGEABLE

OTHER DEPARTMENTS AFFECTED/USERS   1._____

2._____

3._____

4._____

5._____

REQUEST FOR ITEM ADDITIONS TO/
DELETIONS FROM/CHANGES TO STOREROOM INVENTORY (cont.)

REASON FOR REQUEST _____

_____

ITEM(S) TO BE REPLACED _____ STOCK # _____

CURRENT STOCK
WILL BE ☐ USED BY DEPARTMENT ☐ RETURNED TO VENDOR ☐ OTHER

STOCK # _____ BASIC UNIT _____ ORDER QUANTITY _____

REORDER POINT CRITICAL LEVEL _____

☐ APPROVED
☐ REJECTED _____ DATE _____
                      (PURCHASING MANAGER)

☐ APPROVED
☐ REJECTED _____ DATE _____
                      (DISTRIBUTION MANAGER)

☐ APPROVED
☐ REJECTED _____ DATE _____
                (DIRECTOR OF MATERIALS MANAGEMENT)

COMMENTS _____

_____

_____

_____

_____

_____

Subject	Effective Date 1-90	Latest Revision & Date
COMPUTERIZED INVENTORY CONTROL SYSTEM OVERVIEW		

The computerized inventory control system (CICS) is designed to provide timely and accurate data regarding the conditions of all "official" inventory items maintained on a perpetual inventory system. It is linked with the accounting system for general ledger, accounts payable, and budget management.

The computer system provides at least a daily update of conditions based on all inventory transactions. Updates may also be available through inquiries.

The system provides this basic information:

1. Current <u>on-hand balance</u>, dollar values, and physical quantities
2. Items and quantities to be ordered to maintain adequate inventory on hand
3. Usage histories on individual items
4. Usage histories and costs for each department (cost center) for budget management

Much other information is available through a variety of reports generated on a scheduled basis or as requested.

Inventory transactions are processed throughout the day both in batches and on-line, based on the need for timeliness and/or efficiency in data entry.

The sequence of processing in batch mode is always:

1. Additions to/deletions from/changes to master file
2. Corrections or adjustments
3. Purchases on order
4. Receipts
5. Returns to stock
6. Issues
7. Returns to vendors

Because of the importance of data integrity and the speed with which the computer system processes the data, absolute accuracy is mandatory. Without a high level of accuracy, the information provided is meaningless, and the institution risks critical supply problems.

To maintain accuracy, discrepancies or errors that do occur are corrected without delay, according to approved procedures.

Information that is batch processed by the computer and output (reports) from the computer are coordinated by the inventory control clerk. The clerk verifies the accuracy and makes corrections when and where necessary, keeping the manager or director informed through reports or conferences. On-line data entry is made by other materials management staff as work is completed.

Reports and records are maintained on file in materials management for five (5) years and are filed chronologically by department (cost center) numerical sequence.

Affected Departments

Reviewed _____

Subject	Effective Date	Latest Revision & Date
DELEGATION OF RESPONSIBILITY	1-90	

Vice-president of finance/controller:

1. Responsible for the internal audit function, i.e., testing the system to see if it is functioning in accordance with accepted policies and guidelines; measures the reasonableness of actual stock vs. reports; audits controls; spot checks document retention; verifies the expense distribution

2. Authorizes adjusting entries at year's end (physical count vs. general ledger variances); determines write-offs for losses and obsolescence

3. Coordinates external audit

Accounting:

1. Audits to certify to management that inventory records are properly created, processed, and retained

2. Links the inventory system with the accounts payable and general ledger systems

Data processing:

1. Processes batched inventory data in a rapid, accurate, controlled manner
2. Distributes reports and returns source documents
3. Certifies to management that entries are made
4. Coordinates inquiries between the institution and the computer system vendor
5. Guides operating staff through direct on-line data entry processes and procedures

Materials management:

1. Purchasing
   a. Creates documents using accurate item number, vendor, purchase order number, unit of measure, and price
   b. Verifies the open purchase order file against the system reports to find obsolete open purchase orders
2. Receiving
   a. Receives stock and accurately records quantity received
   b. Audits the receipt against the purchase order
   c. Assigns the receiving report control number
3. Distributing
   a. Accurately processes requisitions or returns of departmental supplies in accordance with approved policies and procedures
4. Management
   a. Independently manages the inventory system information and document flow; verifies processing; and files documents
   b. Verifies accuracy of inventory reports; makes all necessary corrections
   c. Recommends adjustments, after investigation/analysis, to the vice-president of finance

Affected Departments

Reviewed _____

Page 1 of 1

Subject		Effective	Latest
INVENTORY DATA ENTRY		Date 1-90	Revision & Date

All inventory transactions must be reviewed and prepared for data entry. Some entries are made in batches. Others are made on-line.

The inventory control clerk will review all batch transactions by type. As indicated, items are batched and sorted in the following manner:

1. Master file additions, deletions, changes: computer inventory control complete load/change form
2. Corrections/adjustments: adjustment forms
3. On-orders: purchase orders
4. Receipts: receiving reports
5. Returns to stock: credit reports
6. Issues: stock requisitions
7. Returns to vendors: outgoing report

NOTE: Each cost center will constitute the start of a new batch of issues.

Batches must include the following information:

1. Date
2. Batch control header form (this form identifies the type of transaction for the batch, i.e., issues, receipts, etc.)
3. Batch number:
    Sun. 1-199
    Mon. 2-299
    Tues. 3-399
    Wed. 4-499
    Thurs. 5-599
    Fri. 6-699
    Sat. 7-799
    Sun. 8-899
4. Total line items
5. Total quantity
6. Total cost

All above totals are double-checked on a calculator for accuracy. The tapes are attached to the batch.

All batches are returned to the inventory control clerk for filing and retained there for audit purposes for five (5) years. The batches are filed in numerical, chronological order.

After the documents have been entered, they are stamped POSTED: Inventory Control and dated to show they have been processed in case a lost document shows up. The inventory control clerk stamps the documents and files them until they clear, or for no more than 30 days (the beginning of the next calendar month).

On-line data entry is made directly into the computer system files as they occur in purchasing, receiving, and distributing. Hard-copy documentation/source documents are saved as are batch processed documents.

Affected Departments

Reviewed _____

Page 1 of 1

Subject	Effective Date	Latest Revision & Date
REQUESTING REPORTS	1-90	

Some reports in the CICS are not automatically generated and must be requested.

Requests for reports are prepared and submitted to the inventory control clerk. Routine reports should be carefully reviewed to avoid needless preparation of a custom report.

The inventory control clerk will prepare or request reports. Reports are printed as one-, two-, or four-part forms.

When reports are printed or received, they will be disseminated by the inventory control clerk.

Reports received on a regular basis are distributed as follows:

Daily—routine reports

1. Control analysis	Director of materials management, vice-president of finance, inventory control clerk
2. Transaction report	Inventory control clerk
3. Error list	Director of materials management, inventory control clerk
4. General ledger entry	Accounting, director of materials management
5. Action list	Purchasing, inventory control clerk
6. On hand	Purchasing, inventory control clerk, dispatch

Daily—requests

1. See requests for reports above	Inventory control clerk
2. Going-to orders	Purchasing, distribution manager

Monthly

1. Stock status	Director of materials management, accounting
2. Department usage	Director of materials management, accounting, all departments
3. Item status	Director of materials management, purchasing, distribution manager

Annual
1. Usage history	Purchasing, distribution manager

Affected Departments

Reviewed _____

Subject	Effective Date 1-90	Latest Revision & Date
INVENTORY CLASSIFICATIONS		

The following is a list of item classifications by asset class and prefix class, with the description of each classification.

Asset class:

1. Dietary/kitchen supplies
   11—China
   12—Flatware
   13—Miscellaneous kitchenware
   15—Formula
   17—Canned goods
   18—Dry food goods
   19—Paper/plastic cups, utensils

2. Housekeeping (cleaning) and laundry supplies
   21—Cleaning agents
   22—Housekeeping utensils
   23—Paper/plastic bags
   24—Miscellaneous paper/plastic goods
   25—Bed linen
   26—Disposable linen
   29—Maintenance supplies

3. Laboratory miscellaneous
   31—Laboratory solutions
   32—Laboratory glassware and reagents
   33—Miscellaneous laboratory supplies

4. Ancillary supplies
   41—X-ray supplies
   42—Cardiovascular
   43—Respiratory-pulmonary

5. IV fluids
   62—IV fluids
   63—IV sets

6. Medical and surgical supplies
   65—Irrigation fluids
   66—Dressings, tape
   67—Catheters
   68—Gloves
   69—Sterile wrapping material
   70—Orthopedic supplies
   71—Medical gases
   72—Sutures
   73—Needles, surgical
   74—Needles, hypodermic
   75—Syringes, disposable
   76—Trays, kits, and packs
   77—Tubes, tubing, and accessories
   78—Electrical medical supplies (ECG)
   79—Miscellaneous medical and surgical supplies

7. Office supplies
   90—Office supplies and nonprinted paper goods

8. Printed forms and stationery
   91—Printed forms
   92—Stationery, envelopes

Numbering system:

The inventory numbering system is composed of a seven-digit number for each line item in inventory (e.g., 90-07653).

The first two digits identify the class of items, i.e., dietary, linen, etc. (See previous list of categories.)

The next three digits are the item's specific number. The last digit is a check digit, used for data entry purposes. The check digit is used to prevent transposition errors when the item number is processed.

Affected Departments

Reviewed _____

Page 1 of 1

Subject	Effective Date	Latest Revision & Date
PURCHASE ORDERS	1-90	

Purchases for inventory items are generated in the purchasing office on a purchase order form. (See sample.)

Copies of the purchase order are disseminated according to the procedures listed for purchasing stock (inventory) items.

Purchase orders are entered on-line by the buyers.

The information required for data entry is:

1. Total line items ordered
2. Total units ordered
3. Vendor
4. Vendor number
5. Item number
6. Item quantity
7. Unit of measure
8. Unit price
9. Extended cost
10. Contract reference number
11. Required receipt date

This information is accumulated and entered into the computer system as orders are prepared. Hard copies of documents/transactions are maintained only for special orders.

Corrections, additions, and deletions on any purchase orders are made on the computer by the buyer.

The computer system's daily transactions report is analyzed each day by the inventory control clerk to make sure that all transactions have been entered. These reports and records are filed in chronological order and retained for 30 days (the beginning of the next calendar month).

NOTE: The system will accept only two (2) open purchase orders for any line item (even if from separate vendors). To avoid a rejected entry, at least one of the open purchase orders will have to be received or canceled.

Affected Departments

Reviewed _____

PURCHASING ORDER

TO:

TAX EXEMPTION

THE HOSPITAL IS EXEMPT FROM STATE SALES TAX. THE TAX EXEMPT NUMBER IS:

☐ IF X'ED, THIS IS A CONFIRMING ORDER — DO NOT DUPLICATE —

DATE	VENDOR NO.

F O B · HOSPITAL

DELIVERY DATE	SHIP VIA	INVOICE TERMS

SHIP ON OR BEFORE

FOR HOSPITAL USE ONLY

DATE	DATE	DATE
REC'D BY	REC'D BY	REC'D BY
DEPT. SIG.	DEPT. SIG.	DEPT. SIG.

ITEM NO	QUANTITY	PURCH/SHIP UNIT	DESCRIPTION	UNIT PRICE	EXTENDED PRICE	HOSP. ITEM # COST. CENTER #	QUANTITY	DISPENSING UNIT	DISPENSING UNIT COST	QTY. REC'D	QTY. REC'D	QTY. REC'D
1												
2												
3												
4												
5												
6												
7												
8												
9												
10												
11												
12												
13												
14												

SAMPLE

DIRECTOR OF PURCHASING

INV. TOTAL LINE ITEMS ORDERED

INV. TOTAL LINE ITEMS REC'D

☐ ORDER COMPLETE

PURCHASING DEPT. COPY

Subject	Effective Date	Latest Revision & Date
VENDOR RETURNS	1-90	

Inventory items are returned to the vendor for a variety of reasons:

1. Incorrect item shipped
2. Incorrect quantity shipped
3. Double shipment
4. Damaged goods
5. Product recall

In each of these situations, the goods are pulled from their storage area and placed in a holding area in the storeroom.

An outgoing report is prepared by the purchasing staff. (See Returns of Purchased Items, Procedure #2.21.) Copies are distributed to:

1. Vendor
2. Accounting
3. Purchasing
4. Receiving

On completion of the outgoing report (when the goods are technically no longer available for use), the inventory control clerk prepares the "reverse" receiving report (see sample) that will reduce the inventory quantity on hand via a "return" transaction.

The items being returned are deducted from the computer inventory balance by a reverse receipt transaction. That is, a negative quantity is entered along with:

1. Item number
2. Quantity to be subtracted from on-hand balance
3. Unit of issue
4. Total price of the item(s)
5. Notation "order complete"
6. Vendor number
7. Total line items
8. Total units

All returns are reviewed and prepared for data entry. Transactions are entered in the computer system by the inventory control clerk.

The transaction is verified the following day by reviewing the computer system's daily transactions report.

Affected Departments

Reviewed _____

Page 1 of 1

Procedure #3.9

RECEIVING REPORT

SHIP TO   BILL TO:

PURCHASE ORDER NO.

TAX EXEMPTION
THE HOSPITAL IS EXEMPT FROM STATE SALES TAX. THE TAX EXEMPT NUMBER IS:

☐ IF X'ED, THIS IS A CONFIRMING ORDER – DO NOT DUPLICATE –

DATE	DATE	DATE
REC'D BY	REC'D BY	REC'D BY
DEPT. SIG.	DEPT. SIG.	DEPT. SIG.
QTY. REC'D.	QTY. REC'D	QTY. REC'D

DATE

VENDOR NO

TO:

FOB - HOSPITAL

DELIVERY DATE   SHIP VIA   INVOICE TERMS

SHIP ON OR BEFORE

FOR HOSPITAL USE ONLY

ITEM NO.	QUANTITY	PURCH/SHIP UNIT	DESCRIPTION	UNIT PRICE	EXTENDED PRICE	HOSP. ITEM # COST. CENTER #	QUANTITY	DISPENSING UNIT	DISPENSING UNIT COST
1									
2									
3									
4			SAMPLE						
5									
6									
7									
8									
9									
10									
11									
12									
13									
14									

INV. TOTAL LINE ITEMS ORDERED

INV. TOTAL LINE ITEMS REC'D

DIRECTOR OF PURCHASING

☐ ORDER COMPLETE

CONTROL COPY-RECEIVING

154

Subject	Effective Date 1-90	Latest Revision & Date
RECEIVING		

All receipts of stock items are processed through the computer. Receipts increase the balance on hand for that item both in total quantity units (each, case, box, etc.) and dollar value.

Receipts and receiving report forms require:

1. Item number
2. Quantity received (in units)
3. Unit of measure (how handled by the computer—each, case, box, etc.)
4. Unit cost (price)
5. Total cost (price of a unit × total units received)

The receiving report (see sample) should state exactly how many units are received. These units refer to the way the hospital handles them, not the vendor.

When filling out and processing a receiving transaction:

1. Record the actual quantity received in the hospital's units
2. Forward the receiving report to purchasing for matching with the original (control) copy
3. Enter the receiving transaction in the computer system

The following conditions must be handled properly:

1. Quantity received EQUALS the quantity ordered; this makes the order complete. Total cost equals quantity × unit cost. The "order complete" field is checked, and all hard copies of the receiving report are forwarded to purchasing.

2. Quantity received is LESS THAN the quantity ordered. The units received are noted in the first receiving report column. The CICS multiplies the units received × the unit cost to record the total cost for that partial receipt.

   NOTE: If the quantity received is all that is expected on that purchase order, a notation is made by purchasing in the computer file for that receiving report, and the "order complete" field is checked.

3. Quantity received is GREATER THAN the quantity ordered. On the line printed for that item, the quantity received equal to the quantity ordered is noted in the appropriate receiving report column box.

Affected Departments

Reviewed _____

Page 1 of 1

RECEIVING REPORT

TAX EXEMPTION

THE HOSPITAL IS EXEMPT FROM STATE SALES TAX. THE TAX EXEMPT NUMBER IS:

☐ IF X'ED, THIS IS A CONFIRMING ORDER – DO NOT DUPLICATE –

TO:

DATE	DATE	DATE
REC'D BY	REC'D BY	REC'D BY
DEPT. SIG.	DEPT. SIG.	DEPT. SIG.
QTY. REC'D.	QTY. REC'D	QTY. REC'D

DATE	VENDOR NO

SHIP ON OR BEFORE

FOR HOSPITAL USE ONLY

△

HOSP. ITEM # COST. CENTER #	QUANTITY	DISPENSING UNIT	DISPENSING UNIT COST

DELIVERY DATE SHIP VIA INVOICE TERMS

EXTENDED PRICE	UNIT PRICE

F O B - HOSPITAL

ITEM NO	QUANTITY	PURCH/SHIP UNIT	DESCRIPTION
1			
2			
3			
4			
5			
6			
7			
8			
9			
10			
11			
12			
13			
14			

SAMPLE

DIRECTOR OF PURCHASING

INV. TOTAL LINE ITEMS ORDERED

INV. TOTAL LINE ITEMS REC'D

☐ ORDER COMPLETE

CONTROL COPY-RECEIVING

156

Subject	Effective Date	Latest Revision & Date
ISSUES	1-90	

All issues from inventory are processed through the CICS in a batch mode for efficiency and accuracy. The issues reduce the quantity on hand and charge items to department budget accounts. Issues require: item number, quantity, basic unit, and department number.

All issues must be reviewed and batched by the inventory control clerk before they are entered. This is done several times daily.

Batches require the following:

1. Batch number
2. Total departments (cost centers) charged in the batch
3. Total items (units) issued

The inventory control clerk traces the transactions on the computer system's daily transactions report, stock status report, and the department usage reports to make sure they were processed properly. Any corrections are made by the inventory control clerk, batched, and reentered.

Corrections on issues will be made on the stock requisition form.

All stock requisitions are filed by department name/number in chronological order and retained for 30 days (the beginning of the next calendar month).

Affected Departments

Reviewed _____

Page 1 of 1

Subject	Effective Date	Latest Revision & Date
CREDITS (RETURNS TO STOCK)	1-90	

Returns to stock are handled in the same manner as issues (via batch mode), except that the quantity is added to inventory and deducted from department budget accounts. A credit requires: department number, item number, quantity, and basic unit. It is processed like a "negative" issue.

The department prepares a credit by making out a stock requisition in red pencil or red ink. CREDIT is printed on the top of the form.

All credits are reviewed, then prepared and entered by the inventory control clerk. They are stamped POSTED before filing in department sequence.

Affected Departments

Reviewed _____

Subject	Effective Date	Latest Revision & Date
CORRECTIONS	1-90	

Errors will occur during the processing of inventory transactions. These inaccuracies must be corrected immediately so that all information in the system is up-to-date and accurate.

Corrections also may be made to match the physical inventory on hand with the balance on the computer via the physical inventory transaction procedure. Use of this procedure requires prior approval from and the signature of the director of materials management.

"Corrections" are classified according to one of the following types of errors:

1. Item charged (issued) to wrong department (cost center)
2. Cost center (department) charged for the wrong item
3. Incorrect quantity issued or credited to department (includes dispensing unit errors)
4. Incorrect quantity received on receiving report
5. Data entry errors (quantity, stock number, etc.)
6. Incorrect items on purchase order (stock number, dispensing unit, etc.)

In each case, a source document transaction is used to correct the error. This includes issuing a credit to a cost center for an item charged in error, and then charging it properly on a stock requisition to the correct cost center (department).

If clerical errors are discovered on purchase orders, receiving reports, or issues, they are corrected on the computer file before processing is completed. For errors found during audits, a copy is made of each document with the error before a correction is made and presented to the manager for follow-up with the person who made the error.

These correction transactions are prepared and entered by the inventory control clerk. They are stamped POSTED and filed in department sequence, chronologically, and maintained for five (5) years.

Affected Departments

Reviewed _____

Subject	Effective Date	Latest Revision & Date
ADJUSTMENTS TO INVENTORY	1-90	

Inventory adjustment forms are prepared and processed as necessary. The inventory control clerk prepares these forms and presents them to all parties for authorization. This is done to maintain current, accurate inventory records and purchasing reports. Adjustments are charged to the appropriate expense account.

1. Inventory gain or loss

Discrepancies between physical, or actual, count and computer balance must be reconciled to update information/recorded data.

The inventory control clerk will thoroughly research all activity to find the discrepancy in the line item in question. This includes:

a. Receiving reports
b. Returns to vendor
c. Issues from inventory
d. Returns to inventory
e. Other adjustments

If, after investigation, no specific reason can be given for the discrepancy, the inventory control clerk will prepare the inventory adjustment form. (See sample.) The director will approve, sign, and forward it to the other authorizing parties. The item(s) will be assumed lost through either physical (theft, destruction, etc.) or clerical (addition, keypunch, etc.) error.

2. Obsolescence

Inventory items that are no longer usable due to obsolescence will be discarded, and the inventory account will be adjusted to reflect the change. If a department requests the change, it will be charged. If it is an uncontrollable change, the adjustment account will be charged. Obsolescence is either of the following:

a. Expiration of sterile shelf life (fluids, catheter, etc.)
b. Discontinuation due to update in technology, equipment systems, etc.

In all cases of inventory items being discontinued due to a product or procedure change, the balance on hand will either be used up by the user departments or returned to the vendor before replacement items are purchased. Only as a last resort, when items are absolutely unusable, will they be disposed of or destroyed.

If inventory items are classified as obsolete, the inventory control clerk will prepare the inventory adjustment form (see sample) and, in conjunction with the storeroom supervisor, will see that the proper item and quantity is pulled from stock. They will cosign the form and forward it to the director for approval. It will then be returned to data processing for keypunching. After data entry, the documents are stamped POSTED and filed by the inventory control clerk and retained for five (5) years.

Affected Departments

Reviewed _____

Subject	Effective Date	Latest Revision & Date
ADJUSTMENTS TO INVENTORY (cont.)	1-90	

The mechanics of processing an adjustment to inventory are shown in the following steps.

Adjustments:

1. Error: Computer quantity is less than physical inventory on hand.
   Solution: Plus (+), use inventory adjustment form; adds to inventory balance (not to general ledger)
2. Error: Computer quantity is greater than physical inventory on hand.
   Solution: a. Negative (-) adjustment transaction automatically charges to shrinkage account and reduces general ledger
   b. Charge to shrinkage—issue to a shrinkage account
3. Always check transaction first to see if the originals can be corrected:
   a. Reverse original transaction
   b. Process correction
4. Emergencies: Do not use a purchase order; bypass system and direct expense item(s) to user department.
5. Obsolete: Charge obsolete items to user cost-center shrinkage account.
6. Spoiled/destroyed: Charge to materials management shrinkage account.
7. Correction change to the master file on the "basic unit of measure" requires:
   a. Day 1—balance goes to zero, a negative (-) receipt
   b. Day 2—make change
   c. Day 3—add balance; a dummy (+) receipt
8. Latest cost change:
   NOTE: If the receiving report is processed first (before any other transactions), then this step is not necessary.
   a. Can only be done at zero value
   b. Use only when there is a drastic cost change
   c. Fill out the "latest cost field" of computer load/change form
   d. Enter the two-character institutional code
   e. Enter the seven-digit number for which the adjustment is intended; this must be done the same day
   f. Enter 0000 in the "quantity field"
   g. Enter the difference between the old total value and the new total. Total value is equal to quantity × price. This entry should be made in the space provided for value adjustment; e.g., if there are 10 of an item on hand, and price increases from $4.00 to $4.50, the procedure is as follows:
   $10 \times \$4.00 = \$40.00$ (old value)
   $10 \times \$4.50 = \$45.00$ (new value)
   $\$5.00$ (difference in total value); $5.00 would then be entered
   NOTE: If the new total value is such that it will reduce the total value, a column is available to indicate a credit (a "-" will be entered). If "-" is not entered, the assumption is made to add to total cost.

Affected Departments

Reviewed _____

Subject	Effective Date	Latest Revision & Date
ADJUSTMENTS TO INVENTORY (cont.)	1-90	

9. Value adjustment is a total reevaluation of an inventory item that is on hand. It is used only when quantity is zero or to identify drastic cost changes.
10. Changes on <u>chargeables</u> (including chargeable stock items):
    a. Review and change item master on a computer load/change form
    b. Make same changes on supply charge master list
    c. Determine new cost via cost/price work sheet
    d. Establish a new selling price based on that formula
    e. Process revisions on computer
    f. Revise stock requisition
    g. Revise charge tags
    h. Notify user departments
11. Changes on <u>nonchargeables</u> (including nonchargeable stock items):
    Same as above, except steps b, d, and g are omitted
12. Returns to vendors:
    a. Reimbursement—negative (-) receiving report
    b. Replacement—negative (-) receiving report
    c. When new goods arrive, a plus (+) receiving report is written.
13. Establishing order "units of measure" (U/M):
    a. Determine order U/M
    b. Code computer load/change form with the following:
       (1) Order U/M
       (2) Order/basic conversion
       (3) Reorder quantity
       (4) Latest cost
    c. Forward the form to keypunch
    d. On day of update—withhold purchase orders and receiving reports for items being changed—suggest updating on Saturday
    e. Run new reports:
       (1) Purchasing catalog—three copies each
       (2) Computer whole file item status—three copies each
       (3) Computer-printed bin labels—as needed
    f. Can use basic on-order U/M on purchase orders and receiving reports

Affected Departments

Reviewed _____

Subject	Effective Date	Latest Revision & Date
ADJUSTMENTS TO INVENTORY (cont.)	1-90	

14. Inventory transactions that affect the general ledger:

Type of transaction	General ledger effect
Adjustment (+)	None
(-)	a. Decrease inventory control asset account b. Debit department expense (must supply account number)
Receipts (+ or -)	None

Issue (+)	a. Decrease inventory control asset account
	b. Debit department expense
	   (must supply department number and subaccount
	   number from master file)

(-)	a. Increase inventory control asset account b. Credit department expense
Physical inventory	
(+)	None
(-)	a. Decrease inventory control asset account b. Debit materials management shrinkage account

Affected Departments

Reviewed _____

INVENTORY ADJUSTMENT FORM

Date _____

	Item Description	Item (Stock) #	Dispensing Unit	Quantity Count	Quantity on Computer	Quantity Variance	Explanation of Variance (Type I or Type II)	Account # to be Charged
1								
2								
3								
4								
5								
6								
7								
8								

Prepared by _____   Approved by _____
           (INVENTORY CONTROL CLERK)   (DISTRIBUTION MANAGER)

Approved by _____   Approved by _____
           (ACCOUNTING DIRECTOR)   (DIRECTOR OF MATERIALS MANAGEMENT)

Subject	Effective Date	Latest Revision & Date
YEAR-END PHYSICAL INVENTORY	1-90	

The purpose of physical inventory is to reconcile stock report balances with physical balances on the general ledger. This procedure provides management with the current end-of-the-year status of the value of supplies on hand, the annual turnover rate based on the dollar value of items received and issued, and the dollar and physical balances loss/gain during the past year, based on the annual inventory adjustments documented during the past year.

The objective is to determine whether physical count equals the quantity listed on the records. This represents the past year's inventory plus receipts during the year minus (1) issues charged to user departments, (2) returns for credit, and (3) property disposed of as outdated or unsatisfactory for use.

The inventory is taken at the end of each fiscal year. If periodic (cycle) inventories show accuracy and all items are counted during the year, a year-end count may not be necessary. At the time inventory is taken, no other business transactions will take place so that counting is undisturbed.

The director of materials management will notify all departments in advance when inventory will be taken, so that their needs and orders may be planned accordingly. It is important to plan counting so that patient care activities are not interrupted.

While physical inventories/counts are conducted in all in-house departments that maintain any "material" inventory balance, the only inventories that are reconciled to the general ledger are the storeroom, pharmacy, and food service. This is because those inventories are maintained on the books as current assets until they are consumed (issued to a user department), at which time they become expenses.

Departmental inventories (surgery, radiology, emergency, etc.) are counted and valued to determine if departments are accumulating excessive inventories and to evaluate the effectiveness of the distribution system and the institution-wide inventory management efforts.

1. Preliminary work

   a. Arranging of stock—the stock clerks will be assigned the task of putting the stock shelves and case goods areas in order. Where physically possible, all like stock should be confined to one storage area. Stock on the shelves should be neat and put in an identifiable order so that the package or case label on the item is facing outward.

   b. Physical inventory form—the forms used to take the physical count will be patterned after the computer stock catalog, in numerical sequence. The forms will have the following information:

      (1) Sequential stock number
      (2) Item description
      (3) Unit of issue
      (4) Physical count column
      (5) Unit-of-issue price column
      (6) Extended price column

Affected Departments

Reviewed _____

Page 1 of 3

Subject	Effective Date	Latest Revision & Date
YEAR-END PHYSICAL INVENTORY (cont.)	1-90	

c. Receiving activity on days of actual count—all goods delivered on the days of the count will be held in the holding area and will not be added to inventory until after the physical count. All items received before the count day will be added to and counted in the physical inventory.

All items received after the cutoff time must be stamped AFTER INVENTORY; all documents must be so stamped also. This is done so that these items or documents are not included in the physical count without being processed on the inventory records, or vice versa.

d. Requisition cutoff—because of the detail required in taking physical inventory, all departments and individuals who normally requisition items from stock should requisition their needs before the two-day inventory period. The director of materials management will notify the departments of the inventory. Except for emergencies, any requisition received after the cutoff will not be processed until the count is completed. All requisitions filled before the cutoff will be entered as fiscal-year business.

2. Precount procedures

a. The director of materials management will assign counting teams to areas and schedule the count. One person will count, and the other will record the count.

b. Only one person per team need be experienced with the stock.

c. To check performance, each area of stock will be spot-counted after completion of inventory to the accuracy of the physical count. About 10 percent of the total items counted will be spot-checked by accounting department staff.

d. A floor plan of the storeroom, as well as the procedures to follow, will be given to each count team.

3. Counting procedures

a. The team should begin at the lowest inventory number and work consecutively through the assigned area. No item will be omitted. Switching back and forth, or up and down, will not be permitted. Everything will be counted in sequence.

b. The item description, stock number, and dispensing unit should match the item on the shelf. If there are any doubts, the director of materials management should be contacted.

c. The item should be counted and the count recorded on the forms provided. The count will be recorded in the unit of issue. The unit of issue should be circled on the count sheet to show it was noted.

Affected Departments

Reviewed _____

Subject YEAR-END PHYSICAL INVENTORY (cont.)	Effective Date 1-90	Latest Revision & Date

NOTE: Any items stored in more than one location (bulk and active) should have a notation on the shelf or pallet stating the other location. The team should proceed there to continue the count of that item, add up the total count, and note it in the on-hand column. Entries should be made in pencil. An "X" marked on the shelf label will show the item has been counted.

Every tenth (10th) item counted will be counted twice; once by the counter and again by a spot counter. Both counts should be noted on the count sheet. If the two counts do not match, the director of accounting should be contacted. Another count will be taken to determine the official count and be so recorded on the count sheet.

d. After the assigned location has been completely counted, the director of materials management should be notified. He or she will note this on the team assignment sheet and assign the count team to a new area. Count sheets will be turned in at that time. Counters will count only the areas assigned to them.

e. At the end of the physical count, all counting sheets will be arranged numerically, and copies will be sent to the stock buyer to review all product-unit costs.

4. Postcounting procedures

a. The stock buyer will review each line item's cost.

b. The count sheets, when completed, will be prepared for data entry keypunching as they are released by the director of materials management.

c. All items received during the physical count will, immediately following the count, be received and posted to inventory.

d. All normal business will begin again, as usual, when the word is given by the directors of accounting and materials management.

e. After all extensions are made, the controller will review the results of the inventory with the director of materials management. Any discrepancies between the inventory and the general ledger must be explained and justified in a written report signed by both the director of materials management and the director of accounting.

Affected Departments

Reviewed _____

Page 3 of 3

Subject	Effective Date 1-90	Latest Revision & Date
MONTHLY/PERIODIC INVENTORIES		

Physical inventories are taken periodically to verify that the quantity on hand matches the quantity stated on all records and reports.

If the quantity on hand does not match that on the records, a correction or adjustment must be made to produce an accurate record. The reason for the inaccuracy must be determined so that a concentrated effort can be made to correct the situation.

One portion of the total inventory will be counted each week, on Friday or Saturday. The same procedure for year-end inventory applies, except for the total cutoffs and shutdown. The portion is determined by the distribution manager, in conjunction with the purchasing manager or the director of materials management. During the course of the year, all items will have been counted by this weekly method.

If the counts show the records are accurate, the portion counted may not have to be counted at the fiscal year's end. If the accuracy of the weekly counts is very high (within ± 5 percent), no year-end physical inventory will be required.

This decision will be made by the vice-president of finance and the director of materials management.

Subject	Effective Date	Latest Revision & Date
GROUP CODES	1-90	

All inventory items are given a specific group code that categorizes them by type. Reports generated by the computer are printed in order, alphabetically by group code.

The group codes used are:

A = annual contact items— items purchased on a purchase order for the <u>entire year</u>. The entire quantity is ordered at one time, but shipments are made periodically on an as-needed basis.

D = deleted items—all the items deleted from active stock. They will be kept in the group for the remainder of the fiscal year for review purposes. At that time, they will be removed from the file. An item to be deleted will be immediately placed in group code D, so that it will not be reordered.

S = stock—all the items in the storeroom used on an ongoing basis.

T = temporary—items that are being revised, or that require other action, and should not be reordered until the action or revision is completed (example: change of dispensing units that requires "taking an item to zero balance"). Items are to remain in this group only until the action is completed. From this group, items can go to any other group (A, D, or S).

Affected Departments

Reviewed _____

Subject	Effective Date 1-90	Latest Revision & Date
ROUTING OF INPUT/INFORMATION		

All reports, notices, etc., regarding the inventory control system are routed by the inventory control clerk.

It is the clerk's responsibility to see that all parties concerned, or required, review and initial:

1. Load and changes
2. Requests to add, change, or delete
3. Corrections
4. Adjustments (Note: Only the director of materials management can approve an adjustment.)

This review must be accomplished before the transaction is entered.

Affected Departments

Reviewed _____

Page 1 of 1

SECTION IV

RECEIVING
SECTION IV

Subject	Effective Date	Latest Revision & Date
RECEIVING OVERVIEW	1-90	

The receiving office is open Monday through Friday, from 7:30A.M. to 4P.M. Emergency or badly needed supplies will be received by other materials management personnel after those hours and on weekends. Whenever possible, deliveries from vendors are made on an appointment basis between 7:30A.M. and 1P.M.

The receiving office is responsible for all incoming goods for the entire institution. Pharmacy and dietary products are processed through the receiving department, but those respective departments carry out actual verification, inspection, and documentation of receipt of these items.

All other goods are verified and documented by a receiving report. This serves as authorization for payment.

When the goods are delivered to the user department, the receiving report is signed by authorized personnel to indicate delivery and acceptance. These documents are maintained in the files in receiving.

All receiving documents are recorded in log books, sent to purchasing for posting, and then to accounting to be matched with invoices for payment. Inventory receiving reports go to the inventory control clerk for data entry.

Affected Departments

Reviewed _____

Page 1 of 1

Subject	Effective Date 1-90	Latest Revision & Date
RECEIVING COMMON-CARRIER FREIGHT		

1. On receipt of a shipment from a commercial freight line, the receiving clerk will physically count the number of cartons or verify the weight as shown on the shipping document. At the same time, the clerk will check the items for damage before acknowledging receipt.

2. Any damages should be noted on all copies of the bill of lading (B/L), and a claim must be filed by purchasing within five (5) working days. (See sample.)

3. Any shortage must also be noted on all copies of the B/L.

4. Any B/L noted as short should be held five (5) working days awaiting receipt on a free-astray B/L. The purchase order and all related data should be held in the file bin labeled "problems."

5. Any free-astray B/L should be verified in the same manner as the original B/L that had the shortage noted.

6. Any shortage not recovered in 15 days requires that a claim be filed immediately. All claims are filed through the purchasing office.

7. Any shipment with concealed damage that was not noted on the B/L at the time of receipt must be reported to purchasing immediately. Purchasing will contact a representative from that carrier to inspect the item(s) so a claim can be honored.

8. A B/L marked "prepaid and add" means the freight company billed the shipper for the transportation, and the shipper in turn added the freight charges to the invoice for the merchandise. This type of shipment should be noted on the purchase order by purchasing when the order is typed. The receiving clerk will record the purchase order number, vendor, and date received on each B/L, then record on the purchase order the name of the freight company and the purchase order number, B/Ls will then be forwarded to purchasing daily. Purchasing will be responsible for attaching the B/L to the control copy after the freight bill has been approved for payment.

9. All B/Ls will have the signature of the person accepting receipt, the date of receipt, and any noted discrepancies.

Affected Departments

Reviewed _____

BILL OF LADING

STRAIGHT BILL OF LADING -SHORT FORM- Original-Not Negotiable

RECEIVED subject to the classifications and tariffs in effect on the date of issue of this Original Bill of Lading

FREIGHT SYSTEM, INC.

_____ (Name of Carrier)

Carrier's No. _____

Shipper's No. _____

Date _____

FREIGHT SYSTEM

From _____

At _____

Consigned to _____ (Mail or street address of consignee-for purposes of notification only

Destination _____ State _____ County _____

Delivery Address ☆ _____ (To be filled in only when shipper desires and governing tariffs provide for delivery thereof

Route _____

Delivering Carrier _____ Car or Vehicle Initials _____ No. _____

No. Packages	Kind of Packages, Description of Articles, Special Marks, and Exceptions	*Weight (Sub to Cor)	Class or Rate	Check Column	
					Subject to Section 7 of conditions of applicable bill of lading, if this shipment is to be delivered to the consignee without recourse on the consignor, the consignor shall sign the following statement: The carrier shall not make delivery of this shipment without payment of freight and all other lawful charges.
					(Signature of Consignor) If charges are to be prepaid, write or stamp here, "To be Prepaid."
					Received $ _____ to apply in prepayment of the charges on the property described hereon. Agent or Cashier
					Per _____ (The signature here acknowledges only the amount prepaid) Charges Advanced $

Collect On Delivery | and remit to | C.O.D. Charge to be paid by { Shipper ☐ Consignee ☐ }

$ _____

*If joinery moves between two ports by a carrier by water, the law requires that the bill of lading shall state whether it is "carrier's or shipper's weight."

NOTE-Where the rate is dependent on value, shippers are required to state specifically in writing the agreed or declared value of the property.

The agreed or declared value of the property is hereby specifically stated by the shipper to be not exceeding

_____ per _____

Shipper, Per _____

Carrier, Per _____

Permanent post-office address of shipper. _____

Subject	Effective Date 1-90	Latest Revision & Date
RECEIVING UNITED PARCEL SERVICE DELIVERIES		

When receiving the daily shipment from United Parcel Service (UPS), the following must be done:

1. The label on each package must be checked to be sure it is meant for this institution.

2. Any apparent damage must be discovered.

3. The number of pieces must be counted to be sure count received is the same as the driver's count, before the log book is signed.

4. The log book must be signed.

5. All packing slips should be removed.

6. Formal verification and receipt are accomplished by pulling the respective purchase orders and comparing the good(s) received.

Affected Departments

Reviewed _____

Subject		Effective Date 1-90	Latest Revision & Date
	FILING SYSTEM		

1. Receiving documents are filed in alphanumerical/vendor sequence. There is a separate file for the most commonly used vendors, as well as a miscellaneous file for each letter of the alphabet.

2. There are filing bins for:

   a. Purchasing (completed orders)
   b. Filing
   c. Weekend emergency shipments

3. In the back of each vendor file, the contract, or standing purchase orders, will be maintained.

4. Separate files will be set up for collect freight bills and pending problems.

5. Only authorized personnel (inventory control, purchasing, and receiving) have access to the files. When a purchase order is needed, it must be pulled by one of the above personnel and recorded on the in-out file cards to keep track of all purchase orders.

Affected Departments

Reviewed _____

Page 1 of 1

Subject		Effective Date 1-90	Latest Revision & Date
	FILES PURGING		

1. Any purchase order 60 days or older should be pulled from the files periodically and sent to purchasing for follow-up.

2. Purchasing will check with the ordering department to see if it still wants the merchandise.

3. If the goods are still wanted, purchasing should contact the vendor, obtain expected shipping date, and note it on the purchase order.

4. If the department no longer wants the goods, purchasing should contact the vendor, cancel the items, and note the cancellation on the purchase order.

5. Cancellations require the approval and signature of the purchasing manager.

Affected Departments

Reviewed _____

Subject	Effective Date	Latest Revision & Date
RECEIVING STOCK AND NONSTOCK ITEMS	1-90	

1. Receipt of shipment

   a. As a shipment arrives, the receiving clerk makes sure that the truck is appropriately unloaded.

   b. When the shipment has been delivered, the clerk must check the number of cartons to see that it agrees with the B/L before accepting shipment and so noting by signature.

   c. The clerk must determine which shipment is being received to pull the correct purchase order. If the cartons are not marked with adequate identification, the clerk should check the packing slip.

2. Verification of goods

   a. When the order has been identified and the correct purchase order pulled, the clerk will compare the manufacturer's item number and description of each item with that shown on the packing slip.

   b. Then, the clerk compares the quantity and units received with those shown as shipped on the packing slip. Each item must be checked. The packing slip then must be initialed and dated by the clerk.

   c. Next, the packing slip is compared with the purchase order that shows the "official" amount ordered.

   d. As each "stock" item is checked, the institution's stock number and the date should be stamped on the cartons.

   e. For nonstock items, the user department's account number and the date are recorded on the carton.

3. The receiving report

   a. The receiving report acknowledges official receipt of merchandise and serves as authorization for payment by the accounting department. It is generally a copy of the purchase order.

   b. If the receiving report and invoice do not contain the same information on each item, the invoice will not be paid until the discrepancy is resolved.

   c. After the shipment has been checked, a receiving report is prepared with the following information:

      (1) Date received
      (2) Initials of receiving clerk
      (3) Shipping quantity received
      (4) Quantity received converted to the institution's packaging unit (if inventory item)
      (5) Packing slip number
      (6) An "X" in the box for "order complete" if purchase order is complete

Affected Departments

Reviewed _____

Page 1 of 2

Subject	Effective Date	Latest Revision & Date
RECEIVING STOCK AND NONSTOCK ITEMS (cont.)	1-90	

4. Distribution of documents

After proper documentation has been noted, the following copies should be detached and distributed accordingly, if the order is complete.

a. Stock items:

(1) The original receiving report is detached.
(2) All packing slips, B/Ls, etc., are attached to that copy.
(3) The receiving report is placed in the bin labeled "stock receiving reports."
(4) Reports are forwarded to purchasing every hour for further processing.

b. Nonstock items:

(1) The original receiving report is detached.
(2) Packing slips, B/Ls, etc., are attached to that copy.
(3) The original receiving report is placed in the bin labeled "nonstock receiving reports."
(4) Reports are forwarded to purchasing every hour for further processing.

5. Delivery of nonstock items

a. Receiving reports should be separated by department.
b. Items should be delivered within one working day of arrival. The deliveries will be made at the same time stock item orders are delivered to avoid needless trips.
c. When items are delivered to the department, the person accepting the item is required to sign for it in the space provided in the right corner of the receiving report. This indicates delivery was made to the department.
d. Receiving reports and the goods will not be left in the department unless someone signs for them. The receiving clerk will keep the report and the goods in receiving until someone in the department is available to sign.

6. Delivery of stock items

a. After the items have been verified against the purchase order and packing slip, the clerk records or attaches the inventory number to each case or box.
b. All items are delivered to the storeroom so they can be placed into stock.
c. No signature is required for these items when they are delivered to the storeroom.

Affected Departments

Reviewed _____

Subject	Effective Date	Latest Revision & Date
DAILY LOG OF RECEIVING ACTIVITY	1-90	

Each day's receipts are properly documented on receiving reports. They must also be recorded in the receiving log. (See sample.)

1. The log has the following information:

   a. Date
   b. Purchase order number
   c. Vendor
   d. Truck/carrier
   e. Quantity of goods received (line items, pieces, and pounds, as noted on the B/L or packing slip)
   f. Receiving report number
   g. Notation "order complete" or "order incomplete"

2. This information must be recorded for each receiving report processed.

3. In the column marked "receiving report number," the number of shipments received against that purchase order (1, 2, 3, etc.) is recorded.

4. Then the information at the bottom of the log is filled in:

   a. Total for that day's activity
   b. Name of person who prepared the log

The log is maintained in the receiving report's file.

Affected Departments

Reviewed _____

DAILY LOG OF RECEIVING ACTIVITY

Date _____

	PURCHASE ORDER #	VENDOR	TRUCK/CARRIER	QUANTITY			RECEIVING REPORT #	ORDER STATUS
				LINES	PIECES	POUNDS		
1								
2								
3								
4								
5								
6								
7								
8								
9								
10								
11								
12								
13								
14								
15								
16								
17								
18								
19								
20								
21								
22								
23								
24								

TOTAL RECEIVED FOR DAY:　　　　　　　　RECEIVED BY _____

　　• Orders _____

　　• Lines _____ (the number of different products/items)

　　• Pieces _____ (the number of packages)

　　• Pounds _____

Subject	Effective Date	Latest Revision & Date
BACK ORDERS	1-90	

1. When the amount delivered is <u>less than</u> the amount ordered, this is considered a <u>back order</u> (B/O).

2. When preparing the receiving report and a B/O exists, the following information must be recorded on the receiving report:

    a. Date received
    b. Initials of receiving clerk
    c. Shipping quantity received
    d. Quantity received converted to the institution's packaging unit
    e. Quantity back ordered (shipping quantity)
    f. Packing slip number

3. After the proper documentation has been noted, the receiving report is detached from the purchase order.

4. All packing slips, freight bills, etc., are attached to that copy.

5. The original receiving report is placed in the bin labeled "stock receiving reports" if inventory items, and in the bin labeled "nonstock receiving reports" if direct items.

Affected Departments

Reviewed _____

Subject		Effective Date 1-90	Latest Revision & Date
VENDOR SHIPPING ERRORS			

1. <u>Shortages</u>

   When the packing slip (P/S) shows more shipped than has been received:

   a. Check the number of cartons shown on the B/L delivered by the common carrier.

   b. If no other error can be found, it is considered a shipping error.

   c. On the P/S next to the item, indicate whatever the shortage is.

   d. On the receiving report, show what and how many were received. The shortage must be noted above the item for accounting purposes. Accounting will assume a receiving error has been made if not informed of the shortage.

   e. After the proper documentation has been made on the receiving report, detach it from the three-part receiving report set.

   f. Attach to the receiving report the P/S, freight bill, etc.

   g. Notify the purchasing department of the shortage, giving it all the necessary information with a three-part speed memo.

   h. Attach receiving's copy of the memo to the other receiving copies and file in the bin labeled "stock receiving reports" or "nonstock receiving reports," whichever applies. After processing, purchasing will forward a copy to accounting with the receiving report.

2. <u>Overshipments</u>

   There are three types of overshipments:

   a. A duplicate shipment; one that has been <u>received</u> previously

   b. One in which the <u>quantity</u> shipped is <u>more than</u> indicated on the <u>purchase order</u>

   c. One in which <u>more</u> is shipped than is indicated on the <u>P/S</u>

Affected Departments

Reviewed _____

Subject	Effective Date	Latest Revision & Date
VENDOR SHIPPING ERRORS (cont.)	1-90	

Type A overshipment—duplication of the quantity ordered

    (1) Check with the purchasing office and buyer responsible for ordering to determine whether the excess goods will be kept or returned.

    (2) If the goods are to be kept, note on the receiving report "overship, will keep per _____ " (name of authorized person).

    (3) Complete and detach receiving report and file in the appropriate bin (stock or nonstock).

    (4) If the goods are to be returned, purchasing will prepare an outgoing report. [See Shipping (Returns) Overview, Procedure #5.1.]

Type B overshipment—quantity received greater than noted on purchase order

    (1) The amount received must be noted on the P/S and signed.

    (2) Notify purchasing of the overshipment with a three-part speed memo.

    (3) If purchasing and the user department(s) elect to keep the goods, purchasing will notify the vendor so an additional invoice can be sent and will correct or issue another purchase order.

    (4) If purchasing elects to return the merchandise, it will prepare the proper paperwork for the item(s) to be returned.

    (5) Notations are made on the receiving report.

Type C overshipment—quantity received greater than noted on packing slip

    See type B.

Affected Departments

Reviewed _____

Page 2 of 2

Subject		Effective Date 1-90	Latest Revision & Date
	MANUAL RECEIVING REPORTS		

1. Manual receiving reports are needed when the complete receiving report set (1, 2, and 3) has been used on previously received partial shipments.

2. Manual receiving reports are used on both stock and nonstock receipts and on standing orders.*

3. Prepare the manual receiving report by transferring all the information on the original purchase order (PO) regarding only the item(s) being received (see sample). Where possible, avoid handwriting by photocopying the unmarked master copy of the receiving report set or printing extra copies on the computer system.

   a. Vendor
   b. PO number
   c. Vendor number (if stock item)
   d. Quantity originally ordered
   e. Ordering unit
   f. Description
   g. Unit price
   h. Stock or department number
   i. Dispensing unit

   Fill in the following information:

   j. Date
   k. Received by
   l. Quantity received (converted if stock item)
   m. Quantity back ordered (if any)
   n. P/S number
   o. An "X" in appropriate box if order is complete

4. Record on the control copy the item(s) received, the date, quantity received, and quantity back ordered, if any.

5. Attach to the second copy of the manual receiving report the P/S, freight bill, etc.

6. Then, place the manual receiving report in the appropriate bin, "stock receiving reports" or "nonstock receiving reports."

7. Forward to purchasing at the appropriate time.

*Standing orders will use extra copies of the original receiving report to eliminate handwriting.

Affected Departments

Reviewed _____

RECEIVING REPORT

PURCHASE ORDER NO.

SHIP TO:

BILL TO:

TO:

TAX EXEMPTION

THE HOSPITAL IS EXEMPT FROM STATE SALES TAX. THE TAX EXEMPT NUMBER IS:

DATE

VENDOR NO.

☐ IF X'ED, THIS IS A CONFIRMING ORDER – DO NOT DUPLICATE –

DELIVERY DATE	SHIP VIA	INVOICE TERMS	F.O.B. - HOSPITAL

SHIP ON OR BEFORE

FOR HOSPITAL USE ONLY

ITEM NO	QUANTITY	PURCH/SHIP UNIT	DESCRIPTION	UNIT PRICE	EXTENDED PRICE	HOSP. ITEM # COST. CENTER #	QUANTITY	DISPENSING UNIT	DISPENSING UNIT COST
1									
2									
3									
4									
5			SAMPLE						
6									
7									
8									
9									
10									
11									
12									
13									
14									

INV. TOTAL LINE ITEMS ORDERED

INV. TOTAL LINE ITEMS REC'D

DATE	DATE	DATE
REC'D BY	REC'D BY	REC'D BY
DEPT. SIG.	DEPT. SIG.	DEPT. SIG.
QTY. REC'D.	QTY. REC'D	QTY. REC'D

☐ ORDER COMPLETE

DIRECTOR OF PURCHASING

CONTROL COPY-RECEIVING

187

Subject	Effective Date 1-90	Latest Revision & Date
STANDING OR CONTRACT ORDERS		

1. All standing, or contract, orders should be handled in the same manner as any other receipt transaction.

2. After the third shipment has been received, extra copies of receiving reports are used.

3. All shipments must be recorded on the control copy in chronological sequence. Use the back side if necessary.

4. All contracts and standing purchase orders will be kept in the file until others are issued to take their place. Contracts are canceled and renewed annually as necessary.

Affected Departments

Reviewed _____

Page 1 of 1

Subject	Effective Date	Latest Revision & Date
RECEIVING EQUIPMENT	1-90	

1. Contract carrier

   a. Obtain the correct purchase order.

   b. If the cartons are not marked with adequate identification, open them to determine contents.

   c. Match the P/S and PO; check off each item as it is unloaded.

   d. At the same time, check for any apparent damages and note them on the B/L before accepting shipment.

   e. Prepare the receiving report by carefully and accurately noting the items received and any items back ordered.

   f. Tag all capital equipment with an institutional property tag __before__ delivery to the department or installation.

   g. Also note the tag number beside each item on the receiving report before it is sent to purchasing.

   h. Send the original receiving report to purchasing and file the other copies accordingly.

   i. If the PO is incomplete, refile it to await further shipments.

   j. If the PO is complete, send it to the purchasing office.

2. Commercial carrier

   Follow Procedure #4.2.

Affected Departments

Reviewed _____

Page 1 of 1

Subject		Effective Date 1-90	Latest Revision & Date
RECEIVING FLOWERS/PLANTS			

Flowers are delivered through the receiving dock between 11A.M. and 5P.M., Monday through Saturday.

When flowers arrive, the florist transports them directly to the patients' rooms (alcove area) via the staff elevator. The delivery person may use the intercom at the receiving dock to obtain the room numbers from the information desk.

If a delivery is necessary when the receiving dock is closed, the dispatcher may be summoned by a buzzer (located in the receiving area).

Affected Departments

Reviewed _____

Subject		Effective Date 1-90	Latest Revision & Date
PHARMACY DELIVERIES			

Pharmacy items are ordered through a PO, as are any other supplies or equipment.

When pharmaceutical items arrive, the PO number is noted on the P/S and the PO is pulled from the open file.

The packages are counted in receiving and compared with the B/L. Many pharmacy deliveries are "inside" deliveries, whereby the truck driver takes goods directly to the pharmacy. In such instances, receiving should note the arrival and the number of packages delivered on the receiving log.

The pharmaceuticals are delivered to the pharmacy for inspection and completion of a receiving report. The receiving report is forwarded to purchasing for further processing.

All pharmacy orders are considered complete as shipped. There are no back orders.

Affected Departments

Reviewed _____

Subject		Effective Date 1-90	Latest Revision & Date
	EMERGENCY ORDERS		

1. Any department (except dietary and pharmacy) that needs an item in an emergency must call purchasing during normal working hours or dispatch after purchasing is closed.

2. Purchasing will notify the receiving office to expect the item and then send the paperwork as soon as possible.

3. When purchasing is not open and an emergency arises, the department expecting the emergency shipment must notify the dispatcher or the manager in charge of the expected emergency delivery.

4. The dispatcher or manager receives the goods, delivers them, or has the person who ordered them pick up the goods.

5. The person who accepts the goods must sign his or her name and note the department to be charged on the P/S.

6. The manager places the P/S in the bin labeled "emergency or weekend deliveries."

7. The receiving clerk sends the P/S to purchasing for the proper paperwork to be completed when the department reopens for business.

8. If deliveries of stock items are received after normal receiving hours and are not needed for distribution, the initialed/dated P/S should be placed in the bin labeled "emergency or weekend deliveries." The items should be left in the receiving area. Appropriate documentation will be completed the next business day.

Affected Departments

Reviewed _____

Page 1 of 1

Subject		Effective Date 1-90	Latest Revision & Date
	RECEIVING BYPASS		

A <u>bypass</u> is something that goes directly to the user department and does not stop in receiving (e.g., service repairs, repair parts, printing).

1. <u>Local pickups and emergency orders</u>

   a. When purchasing has placed an emergency order, the institution's driver will pick up and present the goods to receiving to be processed.

   b. Purchasing must notify receiving of such emergencies before arrival.

   c. Exceptions allowed to bypass receiving are returned to purchasing for handling.

   d. POs may not be typed until after the merchandise has been received in purchasing because of a lack of price information.

   e. Purchasing notifies the user department of arrival, and the items are picked up in purchasing.

   f. Purchasing processes all required documents.

2. <u>Oxygen (bulk and tank)</u>

   a. Bulk oxygen is signed for by purchasing, and a PO is issued and completed in the purchasing office.

   b. If portable tanks are delivered at the same time as bulk oxygen, receiving personnel handle the transaction in the same manner as any routine receipt.

   c. On weekends, the materials management person in charge must check and sign for any deliveries made.

   d. The signed and dated report is placed in the "emergency or weekend deliveries" bin.

   e. The receiving clerk then forwards the report to purchasing to be assigned a PO number and be completed.

Affected Departments

Reviewed _____

Page 1 of 1

Subject	Effective Date	Latest Revision & Date
LABORATORY REFRIGERATED ITEMS	1-90	

If an item is received that requires refrigeration and is not an emergency item, the receiving report can be processed and the item kept in the refrigerator until a delivery can be made.

If the same type item is received over the weekend or after receiving hours, and receiving has no notification from the laboratory of an item being expected, the P/S with the date and name of the person receiving and the note "in refrigerator" should be placed in the bin labeled "emergency or weekend deliveries." The item should be refrigerated until delivery can be made.

Affected Departments

Reviewed _____

Subject	Effective Date 1-90	Latest Revision & Date
ITEMS WITHOUT PURCHASE ORDERS		

If receiving cannot find a purchase order for an item or has not been told of the expected shipment, receiving personnel will not accept the item until purchasing has been contacted.

If the item is for pharmacy or dietary, receiving will check with that department for approval.

Nothing should be received without a PO. Anything received, whether it is a repair, replacement, or a no-cost sample item, must have a PO number. If an item of this nature arrives, the manager should be notified so it can be brought to the attention of the purchasing staff.

Personal packages for physicians or staff are not accepted by/at the hospital. Any such occurrence must be reported to the manager.

Affected Departments

Reviewed _____

Subject	Effective Date 1-90	Latest Revision & Date
LOST PURCHASE ORDERS		

When it has been determined that a PO has been lost:

1. A copy of the goldenrod copy kept by purchasing should be made.

2. Then, a copy of the accounting copy should be made (if any prior shipments have been received).

3. The two copies should be attached and marked "duplicate—original lost."

4. A manual receiving report for the remainder of the shipment should be made, using the accounting copy as the control copy.

Subject		Effective Date 1-90	Latest Revision & Date
	RADIOACTIVE MATERIALS		

1. When a shipment of radioactive materials arrives, packages should be checked thoroughly before accepting shipment.

2. The user department (usually radiology) should be notified of the shipment, and the materials should be delivered _immediately_.

3. The shipping documents should be signed by a staff member in the user department.

4. These items should not be held in receiving, even overnight. Security should be contacted to gain access to radiology or the destination department, and the items should be left in that department after the person in charge has been contacted and instructions for safe handling/storage have been communicated.

Affected Departments

Reviewed _____

Subject	Effective Date 1-90	Latest Revision & Date
DIETARY DELIVERIES		

1. All dietary deliveries must be channeled through receiving. Dietary deliveries are usually "inside" deliveries—truck drivers take goods directly to the kitchen.

2. Receiving personnel (or dispatchers) are responsible for directing the food vendors through the department to dietary.

3. All receiving reports are prepared by dietary personnel.

Subject		Effective Date 1-90	Latest Revision & Date
	FILING DAMAGE CLAIMS		

When an item is damaged during shipment, the shipper, vendor, and purchasing office must be notified in writing.

If damage is noticeable <u>at the time</u> the goods are received, the type of damage and quantity of the goods involved are so noted on the B/L. This is marked so that the purchasing office will note the situation when the receiving report is processed.

If the damage is noticed <u>after</u> the goods have been received, purchasing must be notified in writing. The type, quantity, and damage information must be noted and forwarded to purchasing.

Purchasing will obtain a claim form from the shipper/vendor and complete it. A copy of the claim form will be kept with the original PO, and another copy will be sent to accounting. The PO is considered open (kept in the open file) until the claim has been resolved.

Affected Departments

Reviewed _____

SECTION V

SHIPPING
SECTION V

Subject	Effective Date	Latest Revision & Date
SHIPPING (RETURNS) OVERVIEW	1-90	

The return of goods and shipping function are the responsibilities of receiving personnel. All items leaving the institution must be properly documented and authorized before shipment or pickup.

When the purchasing office has prepared the necessary documents to return merchandise, it notifies the receiving staff to pick up the items from purchasing or from the user department, as needed.

The items are properly packed and labeled, and the information is logged on the appropriate records. The mode of transportation is selected, and the merchandise is sent.

After the shipment has been picked up, all documents are distributed to their assigned destinations.

Affected Departments

Reviewed _____

Page 1 of 1

Subject		Effective Date 1-90	Latest Revision & Date
	OUTGOING REPORT		

1. Any merchandise to be shipped from the institution must be authorized by purchasing. The documents required to return or ship goods are: bill of lading (B/L), outgoing report, authorization, and shipping label.

2. Purchasing will prepare three copies of the outgoing report (see Returns of Purchased Items) and shipping labels and notify receiving that it has items to be shipped. (See sample.)

3. The only exception to the above is when the items (stock and nonstock) are being returned by receiving due to a shipping error. Then, a request for an outgoing report will be prepared by receiving, with the necessary information needed to prepare the report.

4. Receiving will not accept any outgoing shipments without the necessary documentation.

5. Purchasing retains the yellow copy of the outgoing report and attaches it to the goldenrod copy of the corresponding purchase order (PO).

6. The pink copy is forwarded to accounting to inform that office not to pay any invoice for the item(s) noted for return, or to expect a credit memo.

7. The white copy is sent to receiving to be used as the packing slip (P/S).

8. If the goods are going to be replaced, no copy is sent to accounting; the pink copy is sent to receiving to notify its personnel of the expected replacement.

Affected Departments

Reviewed _____

OUTGOING REPORT

IMPORTANT!

THE REFERENCE NUMBER LISTED BELOW MUST APPEAR ON ALL PACKAGES, SHIPPING PAPERS, INVOICES, CREDITS AND OTHER CORRESPONDENCE

REFERENCE NUMBER

THE REASON FOR SHIPMENT OF THE ITEMS LISTED IS:

- [ ] RETURN FOR EXCHANGE
- [ ] LOANED*
- [ ] RETURN FOR CREDIT
- [ ] INCORRECT ITEM RECEIVED
- [ ] SENT FOR REPAIR
- [ ] SALES*
- [ ] RETURN TO LENDER/RENTER
- [ ] OTHER*

* HOSPITAL is absolved of any liability resulting from the use of any items lent or sold

DATE:

SHIPPED VIA: _____ CARRIER _____

_____ / PREPAID OR COLLECT

[ ] DELIVERED [ ] PICK-UP [ ] OTHER

ITEM NUMBER	QUANTITY	UNIT	PRODUCT NO.	DESCRIPTION	UNIT PRICE	AMOUNT
1						
2						
3						
4						
5						
6						
7						
8						
9						
10						
11						
12						
13						
14						

TOTAL NUMBER OF PIECES

RECEIVED BY _____ OUTGOING DATE _____

DRIVER _____

SHIPPING CLERK _____ RETURN DATE _____ **PACKING LIST**

Subject		Effective Date 1-90	Latest Revision & Date
	PACKING AND LABELING		

1. The outgoing goods must be securely packaged to avoid damage during shipment.

2. A copy of the outgoing report, and any other return-goods authorizations that may be required, should be placed inside the package. Then, the package is sealed.

3. The shipping label is placed on the outside of the carton where it can be seen easily.

Affected Departments

Reviewed _____

Subject	Effective Date	Latest Revision & Date
SHIPPING DOCUMENTS	1-90	

1. United Parcel Service (UPS)

   a. After it has been boxed and labeled, the package must be stamped with the UPS stamp bearing the institution's identification number and the weight blank.

   b. The package must be weighed, and the weight logged in the space on the package. UPS has a total weight limit per package.

   c. Then, from the outgoing report copies, the required information should be written in the UPS pickup book.

   d. In the outgoing report "reference number" box, the report number, or the PO number should be written if the item is being sent out for repair or replacement.

   e. The company name, street address, city, state, and zip code should be filled in.

   f. The weight of the package and the zone to which it is being shipped should both be recorded in the appropriate space.

   g. The zone (2 through 8), found on the UPS zone chart, is determined by the first three digits of the zip code. For example, if the destination's zip code is 53526, the zip code prefix is 535 and the destination is zone 5.

   h. If the package is to be insured for a value of more than $100, the declared value must be written on the line below the address.

   i. After this information has been recorded in the UPS pickup book (see sample), the UPS page number should be written on the outgoing report.

   j. The information needed should be recorded on the shipping log.

2. Common-carrier freight lines

   a. Any item over 50 pounds, not requiring insurance for a value of more than $1,000, can be returned by common carrier.

   b. The procedures for packing and labeling should be followed.

   c. The shipping documents should be prepared according to the following sample.

   d. The B/L should be marked "prepaid" or "collect."

Affected Departments

Reviewed _____

SAMPLE ENTRIES IN UPS PICKUP RECORD

[4] United Parcel Service
UPS PICKUP RECORD

Customer's check accepted at shipper's risk unless otherwise noted on C.O.D. tag

UPS COPY

STAMP YOUR UPS SHIPPER NUMBER HERE

1-23-456

EXAMPLE FROM TERRITORY SERVED ZONE CHART (40 01 TO 141 99)		
ZIP CODE PREFIX		ZONE
120 — 129		3
130 — 132		2
133 — 135		3
136 — 149		2

NY
S.— 1213

SALES MEMO	NAME	STREET	CITY	STATE	ZIP CODE	INIT.	WEIGHT BY ZONE							C.O.D. AMOUNT
DATE							2	3	4	5	6	7	8	
PAID OR CHARGE (for 11 lb. 2 oz. package, show weight as 12 lbs.)														
1227	JOHN JONES & Co.	478 ATLANTIC AVE.	HASTINGS	N.Y.	13076	12								
COD (fill out UPS COD tag and attach over address label)														
1249	JOE SMITH, INC.	500 WEST LAKE ST.	COOPERSTOWN, N.Y.		13326	15								12.98
DECLARED VALUATION IF IN EXCESS OF $100 (Show total declared value on line below address)														
1263	FRANK & Co.	222 EAST JACKSON Ave.	NAPLES	N.C.	28760	9								VALUE
		DECLARED VALUE $327.00												
CALL (Fill out separate UPS call tag for each package to be picked up, show weight on call tag)														
1270	JONES & SMITH	111 HARTFORD ST.	DOWNEY	PA.	15530	7								CALL
OVERSIZE (Over 84 inches in length and girth combined, enter actual weight and show "OS")														
1277	ADAMS & Co.	1128 BROADWAY	LAMONT	TENN.	37172	10								O.S.

YOUR COMPANY
YOUR ADDRESS
YOUR CITY, STATE & ZIP CODE

PLEASE DO NOT WRITE ANYTHING IN THE LOWER RIGHT SECTION OF THE PICKUP RECORD.

THIS IS RESERVED FOR OPTICAL SCANNING

UPON RECEIPT OF SUPPLIES PLEASE STAMP YOUR SHIPPER NUMBER ON: EACH PAGE OF THE PICKUP RECORD, ON EACH C.O.D. TAG, AND ON EACH CALL TAG.

208

BILL OF LADING

STRAIGHT BILL OF LADING -SHORT FORM- Original-Not Negotiable

RECEIVED subject to the classifications and tariffs in effect on the date of issue of this Original Bill of Lading

Carrier's No. _____

Shipper's No. _____

Date _____

FREIGHT SYSTEM, INC.

_____ (Name of Carrier)

FREIGHT SYSTEM

From _____

At _____

[paragraph of small print terms and conditions]

Consigned to _____

(Mail or street address of consignee for purposes of notification only)

Destination _____ State _____ County _____

Delivery Address *
(To be filled in only when shipper desires and governing tariffs provide for delivery thereof)

Route _____

Delivering Carrier _____ Car or Vehicle Initials _____ No. _____

No. Packages	Kind of Packages, Description of Articles, Special Marks, and Exceptions	*Weight (Sub to Cor.)	Class or Rate	Check Column	
					Subject to Section 7 of conditions of applicable bill of lading, if this shipment is to be delivered to the consignee without recourse on the consignor, the consignor shall sign the following statement:
					The carrier shall not make delivery of this shipment without payment of freight and all other lawful charges.
					_____ (Signature of Consignor)
					If charges are to be prepaid, write or stamp here, "To be Prepaid"
					Received $ _____ to apply in prepayment of the charges on the property described hereon.
					Agent or Cashier
					Per _____ (The signature here acknowledges only the amount prepaid)
					Charges Advanced $ _____

Collect On Delivery | and remit to _____

$ _____

C.O.D. Charge
to be paid by { Shipper ☐   Consignee ☐ }

** _____ shipment moves between two ports by a carrier by water, the law requires that the bill of lading shall state whether it is "carrier's or shipper's weight."

NOTE-Where the rate is dependent on value, shippers are required to state specifically in writing the agreed or declared value of the property.

The agreed or declared value of the property is hereby specifically stated by the shipper to be not exceeding

_____ per _____

Shipper, Per _____

Carrier, Per _____

Permanent post-office address of shipper _____

Subject	Effective Date 1-90	Latest Revision & Date
SHIPPING LOG		

1. From the outgoing report copies remaining, the following information should be transferred to the shipping log (see sample):

   a. Company name
   b. Outgoing report number
   c. Department returning the goods
   d. Description of items being returned
   e. Quantity of goods being returned, including line items, pieces, and weight
   f. Reason for return (credit, replacement, or repair)
   g. Date returned to vendor
   h. Shipping B/L number
   i. Shipped via (type of service)
   j. Initials of shipping clerk

2. After the information has been recorded on the shipping log, the appropriate copies of any documentation should be forwarded to their destinations.

Affected Departments

Reviewed _____

SHIPPING LOG

| COMPANY NAME | OUTGOING REPORT # | DEPARTMENT RETURNING | QUANTITY | | ITEM(S) SHIPPED | RETURN REASON | SHIPPING DATE | SHIPPED VIA | B/L NUMBER | SHIPPING CLERK |
			LINES	PIECES	WEIGHT						

Subject	Effective Date 1-90	Latest Revision & Date
RETURN OF REPAIRS AND REPLACEMENTS		

1. When an item requiring repair has been picked up from purchasing, it must be accompanied by a PO and an outgoing report.

2. Procedures for packing and labeling should be followed, and the mode of transportation should be determined.

3. When an item requiring repair is to be picked up by a vendor, the item and documentation will be obtained from purchasing.

4. Information from the documentation must be recorded on the shipping log.

5. When the vendor picks up the items and PO, he or she signs the shipping log.

Affected Departments

Reviewed _____

SECTION VI

SUPPLY STORAGE
SECTION VI

Subject	Effective Date	Latest Revision & Date
STOREROOM OVERVIEW	1-90	

The storeroom is the primary location of all stock supplies used throughout the institution. All items must be maintained in a clean, neat, and orderly manner that maximizes space and staff productivity and facilitates maintaining accurate inventory records and filling customer orders.

The storeroom will be kept clean. The floors should be swept daily and scrubbed/mopped as scheduled.

The shelves, bins, etc., that contain supplies must be kept clean, free of dust, dirt particles, and paper trash. Floors should be free of trash.

All aisles should be kept clear. Empty boxes should be removed immediately.

All cartons with "UP" side marked should be stored accordingly. All items should be stored with labels facing front and stacked evenly.

All items should be stored 6 inches off the floor, especially disposable and sterile medical and surgical supplies.

Sprinkler heads must be unobstructed. Items must be stored 18 inches below the sprinkler heads.

Affected Departments

Reviewed _____

Subject		Effective Date 1-90	Latest Revision & Date
STOREROOM LAYOUT			

1. The storeroom is the central storage location for supplies that are used regularly.

2. Storeroom items are cataloged by asset class or category and are placed, as much as possible, in numerical sequence, according to inventory number.

3. There are three basic types of storage in the storeroom:

    a. The small shelving is for small items.

    b. The large shelving is for bulkier items.

    c. The pallet section holds the larger, hard-to-handle items and items with high-volume usage.

4. The storeroom's layout is planned for maximum space utilization and for efficient receiving, storing, and issuing of supplies.

    a. Aisles are maintained to handle the flow of traffic and the material-handling vehicles used. Row aisles should be 1.5 times the width of the largest cart/vehicle used.

    b. Labels are placed on each aisle, section, and item stored. This provides a specific location for every item.

        (1) Aisles are labeled alphabetically (A, B, C), with the appropriate sign.

        (2) Sections are labeled numerically (1, 2, 3). Each aisle has many sections labeled like street addresses (<u>even</u> on the right, <u>odd</u> on the left). This further aids in locating items, even if numerical (by product number) sequence is used.

        (3) Shelves are labeled alphabetically (a, b, c, etc.) starting with the bottom shelf going up. This further defines the location. For example, an item's location may be aisle <u>A</u>, section <u>13</u>, shelf <u>d</u>).

        (4) Item labels on every item stored include the following:

            (a) Item stock number
            (b) Item description
            (c) Unit of measure (issue)
            (d) Reorder point level

        Shelf labels are placed on the shelf edge directly below the item location, except for items on the bottom "a" shelf. Labels for these are on the edge of the shelf above, but set slightly below the labels for items on shelf "b," so that the difference is obvious.

Affected Departments

Reviewed _____

Subject	Effective Date	Latest Revision & Date
STOREROOM LAYOUT (cont.)	1-90	

c. Location sequence is generally numerical by institutional inventory/product number. The location (address) is noted on the inventory records and department locator file for all items stored.

Exceptions to the numerical sequence can occur when:

(1) Different storage modes are required for items in numerical sequence (e.g., IV sets and needles may be stored on small shelving, and IV fluids on pallets—they physically cannot be next to each other). When this occurs, a label for that item is placed in the correct sequence with a note indicating the address/location for the item.

(2) Items stored in large quantities may have two locations; in the issuing section on shelves and in bulk on pallets. Whenever there are two locations for an item, a temporary label is placed next to the bin label with the other location and the date received noted (e.g., A-16-f 7/90).

(3) Items that temporarily need more space than normally assigned also have a dual label (see above) denoting the other location. This may occur when usage of an item temporarily peaks and larger inventories are required, or when a special bulk-purchase discount is offered, or in bad weather months when availability/serviceability or delivery problems dictate large volume purchases and "stockpiling."

5. Space utilization is optimized by loading shelves with product according to the average on-hand quantity required, as determined by demand/usage and inventory turns designations.

a. Items are placed on the shelf in numerical sequence, beginning on the bottom shelf. The average quantity on hand/required is then calculated, and that amount of space is allocated for that item. This continues for all items until the shelf in that section is full. Then, the next shelf up (shelf "b") is positioned so that it is approximately 3 to 4 inches above the top of the product on the shelf below (shelf "a"). This minimizes the gaps or holes and fills the shelf space thoroughly. Generally, the top shelf is "saved" to accommodate overflow.

b. When more of a given item is brought in temporarily, the extra stock is placed on the top shelf in the closest aisle/section to its permanent location, and the appropriate label is placed next to the bin label designating the extra stock's location [see steps (2) and (3) above].

c. Periodically, the storeroom is reorganized and space reallocated to account for additions and deletions as well as quantity/space change requirements.

Affected Departments

Reviewed _____

Subject	Effective Date 1-90	Latest Revision & Date
STOCK ROTATION		

To prevent stock deterioration or expiration of sterile products, the oldest products should always be issued first. Remember: first in, first out. This formula contributes to better patient care and saves money. Generally, all case goods have the date of receipt stamped on them by in-house staff on arrival.

Dated items particularly must be checked by the stock clerk to ensure that the items with the earliest expiration date are issued first. The manager performs a surveillance check at least once a month to verify that the rotation-of-stock procedure is being implemented effectively.

All items that do not have an expiration date should be handled similarly.

Affected Departments

Reviewed _____

SECTION VII

SUPPLY DISTRIBUTION
SECTION VII

Subject	Effective Date 1-90	Latest Revision & Date
SUPPLY DISTRIBUTION OVERVIEW		

Supply distribution, one of the most important functions of materials management, dispenses items in an established unit of measure through the distribution system. Direct purchase items are delivered directly to user departments.

The two types of distribution systems used are:

1. Par restock
2. Departmental requisitions

Both are processed on a scheduled basis according to volume and the needs of in-house departments.

The par restock system provides a 24- to 72-hour supply of items, depending on the user department's needs.

The departmental requisitions are filled, and the items are delivered on the assigned day, usually weekly.

All activity is processed daily through inventory control to keep inventory records updated and to allocate charges for supply items. This is consistent with the perpetual inventory system.

Affected Departments

Reviewed _____

Page 1 of 1

Subject		Effective Date 1-90	Latest Revision & Date
	STOCK CATALOG		

The stock catalog is a numerical sequence listing of all items stored in inventory (physically maintained in the storeroom).

All items are organized in and assigned to an asset class or category. This provides a guideline for the placement and numbering of inventory items. (See Inventory Classifications.)

The catalog follows this format: Item number/vendor/description/dispensing unit.

The dispensing unit is the packaging unit by which the item is priced and issued.

The catalog is updated at least annually and distributed to all departments.

Affected Departments

Reviewed _____

Page 1 of 1

Subject	Effective Date	Latest Revision & Date
DISPENSING UNITS	1-90	

The following is a list of standard two-character abbreviations for dispensing units for the inventory system.

<u>Dispensing Units</u>

1. BC — bag
2. BT — bottle
3. BX — box
4. CN — can
5. CT — carton
6. CS — case
7. DZ — dozen
8. DM — drum
9. EA — each
10. GL — gallon
11. PK — package
12. PD — pad
13. PR — pair
14. QT — quart
15. RL — roll
16. TU — tube
17. VI — vial
18. ST — set
19. JG — jug

These abbreviations will be used for all inventory transactions.

These descriptions include the quantity per each packaging unit (e.g., CS/100, PK/12).

Affected Departments

Reviewed _____

Subject	Effective Date	Latest Revision & Date
DISTRIBUTION SCHEDULE	1-90	

1. All departments order and receive supplies on a schedule that maintains inventories at appropriate levels and balances the workload in the storeroom. Departments submit a properly completed stock requisition to the storeroom no later than 12 noon on the day listed on the schedule. (See sample.)

2. Orders are filled and delivered by storeroom personnel on the following day, usually before 12 noon, so that they can be properly reviewed, accepted, and put away.

Affected Departments

Reviewed _____

Subject	Effective Date 1-90	Latest Revision & Date
DISTRIBUTION SCHEDULE (cont.)		

ALL DEPARTMENTS' ORDERS MUST BE SUMITTED BY 12 NOON THE DAY SHOWN — ORDERS WILL BE DELIVERED THE FOLLOWING DAY BY 12 NOON

MONDAY	TUESDAY	WEDNESDAY	THURSDAY	FRIDAY
751 Laboratory	707 Cardiac diagnostic	701 Nursing service	500 Switchboard	612 Auxiliary/ volunteers
500 Medical staff	605 Electro- cardiogram	611 Social service	759 Housekeeping	500 Administration
603 Medical records	710 Surgery	801 Accounting	758 Pharmacy	610 Pastoral care
703 Emergency room	752 X-ray	803 Business office	757 Respiratory therapy	651 Materials management
712 Recovery room	754 Nuclear medicine	802 Admitting	760 Plant operations	500 Information
606 Catheterization laboratory — special procedures	604 Medical audit	575 Personnel	761 Maintenance	609 Occupational therapy
	756 Pulmonary function			
	714 Discharge planning/ home care	550 Community relations	755 Biomedical electronics	607 Physical therapy
		804 Systems/data processing	601 Dietary	608 Speech therapy

Affected Departments

Reviewed _____

Department	MATERIALS MANAGEMENT		Policy/ Procedure #7.5

Subject		Effective Date 1-90	Latest Revision & Date
	DELIVERY OF ORDERS		

Whenever possible, <u>all orders</u> destined for a user department will be delivered on the same trip. This includes stock orders, nonstock direct orders from receiving, large packages of mail, etc.

1. On delivery to the requesting department, the stock clerk will present the order(s) to the person authorized to accept supplies. That person will inspect the order for accuracy and sign the requisition in the space provided, indicating verification that the items were delivered.

2. Should the department require it, a copy of the requisition(s) will be left with the department for its files or reference. The storeroom will keep and file all originals.

3. To maintain the schedule, orders must be signed for on delivery.

4. The stock clerks then place the copies of all forms/paperwork in the appropriate file.

Affected Departments

Reviewed _____

Page 1 of 1

Subject	Effective Date	Latest Revision & Date
STOCK REQUISITIONS	1-90	

Departments order items from stock according to predetermined quotas or par levels, based on restocking frequency, consumption needs, and sound inventory management guidelines. Materials management assists departments in establishing the levels. These are preprinted on the department's customized requisition as a guide for ordering. They are generated by the computer system based on what has been ordered/issued in the previous 90 to 180 days.

All departments must submit completed, preprinted stock requisitions with the following information:

1. Department name
2. Department number (cost center)
3. Date ordered
4. Signature of authorized department representative
5. Quantity requested in units
*6. Item description
*7. Item dispensing unit
*8. Item stock number

*This information must be furnished when submitting handwritten requests for items. It can be obtained from the stock catalog (issued to all departments).

Requisitions should be completed in blue or black ball-point pen only to facilitate legibility.

All preprinted stock requisitions are set up by asset class (inventory product category) groupings. Each requisition page contains up to 140 line items. Blank spaces are provided for write-in requests.

The preprinted stock requisitions are maintained by materials management. The departments will order these forms as needed.

User department:

1. Fills out requisition
2. Sends the copy to the storeroom on or before the day scheduled
3. Signs the order on delivery

Storeroom:

1. Checks for department name and number
2. Compares ordering unit against dispensing unit
3. Sends the requisition back to the department to be corrected if the requisition is not properly filled out
4. Files it in the appropriate day's bin to be filled if the requisition is correct

Affected Departments

Reviewed _____

Subject	Effective Date	Latest Revision & Date
STOCK REQUISITIONS (cont.)	1-90	

Stock clerk:

1. Fills orders for each day according to the schedule
2. Records amount pulled from the shelf in the "quantity issued" column
3. Records a zero (0) in "quantity issued" column if out of an item being ordered
4. Contacts the manager to check the order
5. Makes corrections if the order is not filled correctly (after being rechecked, it is initialed by the manager or checker)
6. Delivers order to the destination department
7. Contacts the designated personnel in that department to check the order and sign for it (order will not be delivered and left there—someone must sign for it)
8. Returns the signed requisition to the storeroom
9. Places both copies in the basket labeled "filled requisitions"

Affected Departments

Reviewed _____

Subject	Effective Date	Latest Revision & Date
STOCK BACK ORDERS	1-90	

1. When the quantity on hand of an item is found to be below reorder point or zero, it is reported to the distribution manager.

2. The manager contacts the purchasing office to determine the status of the item(s).

3. If the item is unobtainable in a timely manner for reasons beyond purchasing's control, a substitute is obtained after purchasing contacts the user department to discuss acceptable substitutes. For predetermined substitutes, purchasing will proceed and notify the user department that the substitute will be obtained and when delivery can be expected.

4. The user department determines an acceptable substitute, and purchasing obtains the recommended substitute as soon as possible.

5. If the item ordered cannot be obtained and delivered to the requesting department, the stock clerk will prepare a back-order stock requisition for the item(s) and place it in the "back order" bin.

6. The "back order" bin is checked daily, and the orders are filled and delivered as soon as the goods are received. The user department does not need to reorder the item(s).

Affected Departments

Reviewed _____

Page 1 of 1

Subject	Effective Date 1-90	Latest Revision & Date
EMERGENCY ORDERS		

Departments may require stock orders to be processed at a time other than that scheduled. Emergency orders are handled on a first come, first served basis. They are filled after being reviewed and signed by the distribution manager.

The distribution manager and the department manager evaluate such emergencies on an individual basis and attempt to find the cause <u>after</u> the order has been processed, so that emergencies may be minimized.

In the absence of the manager, clerks will fill the order without question as quickly as possible, making sure a requisition form is properly filled out. The matter will be reviewed later by the manager or director. This includes a comparison of par/quota levels to determine the level of adequacy, to avoid frequent emergency orders.

During hours that the storeroom is not staffed, the dispatcher will process emergency orders.

Affected Departments

Reviewed _____

Subject	Effective Date	Latest Revision & Date
CREDITS AND RETURNS (INVENTORY)	1-90	

1. Credits will be handled in a manner similar to stock requisitions.

2. The same form (stock requisition) will be used to _return_ items to stock for credit, except the form will be made out in _red_ ball-point pen.

3. The same information is required on a credit as required on a requisition: department name, number, date, etc. The amount to be returned should be listed in the "quantity ordered" column.

4. The stock clerks will verify the item and quantity, note the exact amount returned in the "quantity issued" column, and stamp <u>CREDIT</u> in red so that the item will not be mistaken for an issue from stock.

5. Credits will be submitted to the storeroom on the same schedule as stock requisitions unless there is defective merchandise that must be returned or replaced. These situations will be handled as needed during normal working hours, following the same procedures used for emergency requisitions.

Affected Departments

Reviewed _____

Page 1 of 1

Subject	Effective Date	Latest Revision & Date
AUTOMATIC SUPPLY DISTRIBUTION SYSTEM	1-90	

All nursing units and many ancillary departments receive their medical/surgical supplies via a par restock system. Quantities of supplies stocked in the departments are predetermined by the user department based on its historical usage.

Par levels are set up to last until the next restock is scheduled. The frequency is determined by user need, space availability, and inventory targets.

Supplies are delivered to the user department at a scheduled time. Items are always placed in the same area for uniformity and ease of location.

The stock clerk or a staff member of the user department takes a complete inventory of the supplies and notes what is missing according to the par levels on the stock requisition (see sample) in the "quantity requested" column.

The clerk determines what is missing by comparing the quantity on hand against the quota shown on the requisition for each item.

The clerk transmits the order/requisition to the storeroom for filling. When the order is filled, it is checked by the manager or another clerk for accuracy, delivered, and put away in the user department.

After they are returned to the storeroom, the forms/documents are routed to data entry and filed appropriately.

NOTE:

1. <u>Inventory</u> and <u>noninventory</u> items that are <u>patient chargeable</u> must have charge tags attached to the item. These items are charged out on the par restock requisition.

2. <u>Inventory</u> and <u>noninventory</u> items that are <u>nonpatient chargeable</u> also are charged out on the par restock requisition but <u>do not require charge tags</u>.

The distribution manager and inventory control clerk periodically check filled requisitions for accuracy.

Errors are corrected before the order is delivered to the user department.

Affected Departments

Reviewed _____

PAR RESTOCK REQUISITION

RADIOLOGY

DEPT. NAME					DEPT. NO.					ORDER DATE			

QUOTA/QTY REQ	ITEM	ITEM NO.	QTY. ISS	DISP. UNIT	QUOTA/QTY REQ	ITEM	ITEM NO.	QTY. ISS	DISP. UNIT	QUOTA/QTY REQ	ITEM	ITEM NO.	QTY. ISS	DISP. UNIT
	DEPT. CHARGEABLES	752			2	WASHKINS	21 00907		BX	4	ARTHROGRAM TRAY DISP. #4325	41 00053		EA
6	SHAVE PREP KITS	76 02055		EA	2	UNIVERSAL CATH TRAY	76 00455		EA	5	DRAPE, STERILE ANGIOGRAM 89 X 90	66 02353		EA
1	TAPE WATERPROOF 1"	65 00458		RL	3	YANKAUER SUCTION	77 01808		EA	5	DISPOSABLE MYELOGRAM TRAYS	41 01259		EA
1	TAPE WATERPROOF 2"	65 00508		RL	1	STRAWS, FLEXIBLE	19 00695		BX	10	ISOLATION GOWNS	26 00534		EA
6	K-5OL EXTENSION TUBING	63 40202		EA	10	E-Z SCRUB IODOFORM	79 03875		EA	10	STERILE GOWNS			EA
12	K-Y LUBRICATING JELLY 5 OZ.	79 05052		EA	3	MELTAWAY BAGS			EA	10	STERILE TOWELS			EA
6	NEEDLE DISP. SPINAL 18 x 3½	74 01003		EA	3	ESOPHATRAST	41 00806		TB	36	SURGEON'S STERILE GLOVES SZ. 7½	68 00346		PR
6	NEEDLE DISP. SPINAL 22 x 3½	74 01409		EA	1	NEO CHOLEX GB STIMULANT	41 01309		BX	6	SURGEON'S STERILE GLOVES SZ. 7	68 00247		PR
12	SYRINGE 3cc DISPOSABLE	75 00051		EA	1	BILO RADIO CONTRA MEDIA	41 00202		BX	36	SURGEON'S STERILE GLOVES SZ. 8	68 00445		PR
12	NEEDLE DISPOSABLE 15 x 1½	74 00005		EA	2	CLYSODRAST BISACODYL TANNEX	41 00301		BX	6	SURGEON'S GLOVES SZ. 6	68 00056		PR
12	NEEDLE DISPOSABLE 19 x 1½	74 00203		EA	30	TAPE MICROPORE 1 x 1¼	65 00367		RL	3	SPONGE, GAUZE 4 X 4 16 PLY STERILE 10'S	66 05653		PK
12	NEEDLE DISPOSABLE 22 x 1½	74 00609		EA	1	SURGICAL MASK 510-N	79 05201		BX	200	SPONGE GAUZE 4 X 4 16 PLY	66 05752		EA
12	NEEDLE DISPOSABLE 25 x ⅝	74 00807		EA	6	500cc .9% NACL IRRIGATION	64 00295		EA	6	SZ. 8 STERILE EUDERMIC GLOVES	68 02011		PR
2	#14 5cc FOLEY CATH	67 01157		EA	4	500cc .9% NACL I.V.	62 01024		EA	6	SZ. 7½ STERILE EUDERMIC GLOVES	68 01914		PR
2	#16 5cc FOLEY CATH	67 01601		EA	100	CUPS PAPER 12 OZ. BARIUM	79 03008		EA	10	BARIUM ENEMA UNITS	79 03354		EA
2	#18 5cc FOLEY CATH	67 01650		EA	1	SURGICAL BARRIER HOODS	79 04568		BX	4	DISPOSABLE URINALS	79 09070		EA
6	CATH ADAPTORS	79 02323		EA	1	DISPOSABLE SURGICAL CAPS NURSE	79 02257		BX	2	#12 5cc FOLEY CATHETER	67 01502		EA
50	SCALPVEIN INFUSION 19GA X 12 INCH	74 03108		EA	100	CUPS PAPER 3 OZ.	79 03057		EA	2	#10 3cc FOLEY CATHETER	67 01452		EA
20	SCALPVEIN INFUSION 21GA X 12 INCH	74 03231		EA	2	CUP HOT STYROFOAM 6 OZ.	19 00190		TB	2	#8 3cc FOLEY CATHETER	67 01403		EA
20	SCALPVEIN INFUSION 23GA X 12 INCH	74 03504		EA	4	KLEENEX	79 08700		BX	25	SHOE COVERS	79 08452		PR
1	PLASTIC SPOONS	19 00646		PK	6	DBL STERILED Y-TYPE BLOOD TUBING 2C2558			EA					
1	1" BANDAIDS	66 00258		BX	20	SYRINGE MONOJECT 60cc SR-500	75 01505		EA					
25	4 X 4 STERILE 2'S GAUZE 12 PLY	66 05455		PK	20	SYRINGE 35cc DISPOSABLE	75 01208		EA					
100	BETADINE SWABS AID	79 08155		EA	12	TAPE, INDEX	79 04311		RL					
50	EXAM GLOVES MEDIUM	68 00833		EA	1	GALLON BETADINE SCRUB	79 01358		GAL					
12	1" ZONAS TAPE	65 00557		RL	1	BETADINE SOLUTION	79 01309		GAL					
1	RADIO CONTRA MEDIA GASTROGRAFIN	41 00855		BX	4	DISPOSABLE BEDPAN	79 40356		EA					
36	PT PREP GI X-RAY	41 01358		EA	6	PLASTIC STERILE BOWL	79 00178		EA					
1	RADIO IV CONTRA MEDIA CHOLOGRAFIN	41 00251		BX	24	UNDERPADS 23 X 24	79 09054		EA					
12	IV TUBING ADMINISTRATION SET	63 00255		EA	6	CYSTO CONRAY 43%	41 00459		EA					
2	3" ACE ELASTIC BANDAGE	70 00250		EA	12	CONRAY 30% DRIP BOTTLES	41 00350		BT					
6	RADIOGRAPHIC EXT. TUBING 30"	77 00933		EA	25	CONRAY 60%	41 00400		EA					
6	RADIOGRAPHIC EXT. TUBING 10"	77 00909		EA	12	EMESIS BASINS	79 01259		EA					
100	ADHESIVE REMOVER	79 00061		EA	6	ELECTRODES	78 00105		PK					
100	ALCOHOL WIPES	79 06704		EA	10	BARIUM ENEMA UNITS DISPOSABLE	41 00103		EA					

CONTROL NUMBER		TOTAL LINE ITEMS	
REQUESTED BY		FILLED BY	RECEIVED BY

SECTION VIII

NURSERVER SYSTEM
SECTION VIII

Subject	Effective Date	Latest Revision & Date
NURSERVER SYSTEM OVERVIEW	1-90	

The end point of the supply distribution system is the Nurserver. This is a cabinet in every patient room (located in the alcove area) that contains all supplies necessary for the care of that patient for a predetermined period of time.

The Nurserver is restocked on a scheduled basis with items basic to the care of each patient. In addition, extra or special items that meet the particular patient's needs are placed here so that they are within easy reach of the nurse. The nurse can thus spend more time with the patient.

The nurse must identify what is needed, and the supply technician must make sure the items arrive at that destination before the needed time.

Affected Departments

Reviewed _____

Page 1 of 1

Subject	Effective Date	Latest Revision & Date
SUPPLY TECHNICIAN SCHEDULE	1-90	

Time	Activity
7—7:15A.M.	Breakfast carts to galley
7:15—7:45A.M.	Equipment rounds
7:30A.M.	Specimens to dispatch
7:45—8:30A.M.	Clean Nurservers
8:30—8:45A.M.	Break for technician #1
8:45—9A.M.	Break for technician #2
8:50A.M.	Return breakfast carts
9—10:45A.M.	Restock/reconcile Nurservers
9:15A.M.	Nourishment carts to galley
9:45A.M.	Return nourishment carts to dispatch
10A.M.	Specimens to dispatch
10:45—11:15A.M.	Lunch carts to galley
11:15—11:45A.M.	Lunch for technician #1
11:30A.M.—12NOON	Equipment rounds
11:45A.M.—12:15P.M.	Lunch for technician #2
11:45A.M.—12:15P.M.	Exchange linen carts
12:15P.M.	Return lunch carts
12:30P.M.	Return nourishment carts
12:15—1:30P.M.	Restock linen in Nurservers
1P.M.	Specimens to dispatch
1:30—1:45P.M.	Receive unit dose carts
1:45—2:30P.M.	Exchange unit dose modules
2P.M.	Nourishment carts to galley
2:30P.M.	Return unit dose carts
2:35P.M.	Return nourishment carts
2:30—3:15P.M.	Stock reminder orders
2:45—3:15P.M.	Count inventory on supply carts and deliver carts to storeroom for filling

Affected Departments

Reviewed _____

Page 1 of 1

Subject	Effective Date	Latest Revision & Date
PATIENT CARE FLOOR ACTIVITY SCHEDULE	1-90	

Time	Activity	Personnel Responsible
6:45—7:15 A.M.	Send up breakfast trays/carts (move to galley)	Dietary Dispatch Supply technician
7:15—8 A.M	Prepare/serve breakfast	Dietary/nursing
7:15—8 A.M.	Trash/linen pickup	Housekeeping
7:15—7:45 A.M.	Equipment rounds	Supply technician
7:30 A.M.	Specimens to laboratory	Supply technician
8—8:30 A.M.	Clean Nurservers	Housekeeping Supply technician
8—8:45 A.M.	Pick up soiled breakfast trays (move to soiled utility cart lift)	Dietary Supply technician
8:45 A.M.	Send soiled breakfast trays/ carts to decontamination	Supply technician
8:30 A.M.	Break for technician #1	Supply technician
8:45 A.M.	Break for technician #2	Supply technician
9—10:45 A.M.	Restock/reconcile Nurservers	Supply technician
9:15 A.M.	Send up nourishment carts to galley	Supply technician
9:45 A.M.	Return nourishment carts to dispatch	Supply technician
10 A.M.	Specimens to laboratory	Supply technician
10:45—11 A.M.	Send up lunch trays/carts (move to galley)	Dietary/dispatch Supply technician
11:15—11:45 A.M.	Lunch for technician #1	Supply technician
11:15—11:45 A.M.	Prepare/serve lunch	Dietary/nursing
11:45 A.M.—12:15 P.M.	Lunch for technician #2	Supply technician
11:45 A.M.—12:15 P.M.	Pick up soiled lunch trays (move to soiled utility cart lift)	Dietary Dietary/supply
11:45 A.M.—12:15 P.M.	Exchange linen carts	Dispatch Supply technician
12:15 P.M.	Send soiled lunch tray/carts to decontamination	Supply technician
12:30 P.M.	Return nourishment carts	Dietary/dispatch
12:15—1:30 P.M.	Restock linen in Nurserver	Supply technician
12:30—1:15 P.M.	Trash/linen pickup	Housekeeping
1 P.M.	Specimens to laboratory	Supply technician

Affected Departments

Reviewed _____

Subject	Effective Date	Latest Revision & Date
PATIENT CARE FLOOR ACTIVITY SCHEDULE (cont.)	1-90	

Time	Activity	Personnel Responsible
1:30—1:35P.M.	Send up unit dose carts	Pharmacy/dispatch
1:45—2:30P.M.	Exchange unit dose modules	Supply technician
2P.M.	Reminder orders due	Nursing
2P.M.	Send nourishment carts to galley	Supply technician
2:30P.M.	Return unit dose carts	Supply technician
2:35P.M.	Return nourishment carts	Dietary
2:30—3:15P.M.	Reminder orders stocked	Supply technician
2:45—3:15P.M.	Count par supplies	Dispatch/supply
4P.M.	Specimens to laboratory	Laboratory
4:30—4:45P.M.	Send up supper trays/carts (move to galley)	Dietary/dispatch Dietary
4:45—5:30P.M.	Prepare/serve supper	Dietary
6—6:30P.M..	Pick up soiled supper trays (move to soiled utility cart lift)	Dietary Dietary
6P.M.	Send soiled supper trays/ carts to decontamination	Dietary
7P.M.	Specimens to laboratory	Laboratory
7—7:30P.M.	Trash/linen pickup	Housekeeping
7:30—8:30P.M.	Put away par level supplies	Distribution
10P.M.	Specimens to laboratory	Laboratory
11—11:30P.M.	Soiled hold room cleanout	Dispatch

Affected Departments

Reviewed _____

Subject		Effective Date 1-90	Latest Revision & Date
	RESTOCKING THE NURSERVER		

Each patient room's Nurserver has approximately 24 to 72 hours of patient care supplies. The types and quantities of supplies are predetermined by nursing and materials management personnel.

The items are restocked according to the schedule by the supply technician between 7:30A.M. and 3P.M.

The supply technician will:

1. Count all supplies in the Nurserver and compare them with the listed quota for each item

2. Restock missing items to the established quota (see typical sample on next page)

3. Reconcile chargeable items and follow control procedure for chargeables

4. Note extra items ordered on the control/anticipation sheet, stock what is available, and obtain the balance later

5. Remove any items in excess of the quota or so noted by the nurse on the control/anticipation sheet; return them to dispatch

Affected Departments

Reviewed _____

Page 1 of 2

Subject	Effective Date	Latest Revision & Date
RESTOCKING THE NONSERVER (cont.)	1-90	

NURSERVER — SECOND FLOOR SURGICAL/ORTHOPEDIC

SHELF ONE (Top)

_____ 1 ea	20 00057 Bath blanket		_____ 1 set	Bedside utensils (1 ea — bed pan, wash basin, emesis basin

SHELF TWO

_____ 2 ea	20 00255 Top sheets	_____ 4 ea	20 00602 Wash cloths
_____ 2 ea	20 00354 Draw sheets	_____ 2 ea	20 00503 Bath towels
_____ 2 ea	20 00206 Pillow cases	_____ 2 ea	20 00552 Face towels
_____ 2 ea	20 00073 Gowns	_____ 2 ea	20 00305 Contour sheets

SHELF THREE

_____ 1 ea	24 00307 Toilet tissue roll	_____ 1 ea	79 03107 Denture cup
_____ 1 pk	24 00356 Paper towel	_____ 1 ea	79 03156 Urine specimen cup
_____ 2 ea	76 00067 Carafe liner	_____ 1 ea	79 02802 Stool specimen cup
_____ 1 ea	79 09104 Mid stream	_____ 1 ea	21 00634 Soap
_____ 1 ea	76 00034 Admit kit	_____ 1 ea	24 00257 Soap dish
_____ 1 ea	76 00069 Carafe with lid	_____ 3 ea	19 00190 Styrofoam cup
_____ 1 bx	79 08601 Tempadots		

SHELF FOUR (Bottom)

_____ 2 ea	24 00208 Bath mats	_____ 4 ea	79 00905 Bedside bags
_____ 2 ea	79 02307 Shower caps		

DRAWER

_____ 12 ea	79 06704 Alcohol wipes	_____ 12 ea	79 02901 Paper medicine cups
_____ 6 ea	79 08155 Betadine swabs	_____ 6 ea	79 00152 Sterile cotton applicators
_____ 2 ea	79 08072 Betadine swabsticks	_____ 2 ea	33 00027 Culturette applicator
_____ 2 ea	79 08092 Betadine ointment	_____ 2 ea	79 08908 Tongue blades, sterile
_____ 4 ea	79 05102 KY lubricant, ind.	_____ 6 ea	19 00695 Flex straws
_____ 8 bx	66 00258 Bandaids	_____ 1 ea	77 00404 Airway
_____ 4 pk	66 05158 2 × 2s, 8 ply	_____ 1 ea	79 42055 Epistick
_____ 4 pk	66 05455 4 × 4s, 12 ply	_____ 6 ea	68 00833 Examination gloves, nonsterile
_____ 1 rl	65 01159 Micropore tape, 1 × 10	_____ 4 bx	79 06258 #2 safety pins
_____ 12 ea	79 02950 Plastic medicine cups	_____ 1 ea	63 01808 IV start pack
_____ 4 ea	75 00051 3 cc syringe	_____ 3 ea	74 00104 18 × 1$\frac{1}{2}$ needle
_____ 3 ea	75 00200 6 cc syringe	_____ 2 ea	74 00302 20 × 1 needle
_____ 2 ea	75 00705 12 cc syringe	_____ 3 ea	74 00401 20 × 1$\frac{1}{2}$ needle
_____ 1 ea	74 03058 19 ga. scalpvein	_____ 3 ea	74 00609 22 × 1$\frac{1}{2}$ needle
_____ 2 ea	74 03207 21 ga. scalpvein	_____ 2 ea	74 00807 25 × $\frac{5}{8}$ needle

SOILED SECTION

_____ 1 ea	75 02701 Red box	_____ 2 ea	23 00200 Plastic bag 15 × 9 × 24 c
_____ 12 ea	23 00507 Bag ties	_____ 2 ea	23 00358 Plastic bag 12 × 18 c

Affected Departments

Reviewed _____

Subject	Effective Date	Latest Revision & Date
RECONCILING SUPPLY CHARGES IN THE NURSERVER	1-90	

1. When restocking the Nurserver or at patient's discharge or transfer, the supply technician must reconcile the charge tags in the Nurserver with the control/anticipation sheet and any leftover supplies.

2. There should be a charge tag present for each chargeable item noted on the control/anticipation sheet if the item is not in the Nurserver.

3. If an item is missing and there is no charge tag present, the supply technician will immediately obtain a tag for the item.

4. If a tag, or item with a tag, or an item without a tag, is found in the Nurserver and not noted on the control/anticipation sheet, the technician will check with the nurses in the area to see if that patient was supposed to have the item. If so, it will be entered on the control/anticipation sheet and reconciled. If not, it will be investigated and charged accordingly.

5. Once reconciliation has taken place, the tags and control/anticipation sheets are taken to the administrative communications clerk's desk for data entry.

6. When reconciling patient discharges or transfers, all extra items are pulled from Nurservers, such as over-stocked needles, syringes, medicine cups, sputum cups, fluids, 4 x 4s, ABDs, partial rolls of tape (paper or adhesive), etc. All items should be returned to stock.

Affected Departments

Reviewed _____

Page 1 of 1

Subject	Effective Date 1-90	Latest Revision & Date
CONTROL OF CHARGEABLE SUPPLY ITEMS		

All patient chargeable items are distributed to their destination with a charge tag already attached.

*This charge tag must be accounted for and processed to charge the patient.

All chargeable items placed into the Nurserver must be noted on the control/anticipation sheet. (See sample.)

The supply technician is responsible for recording chargeable items when restocking the Nurserver or when obtaining a "call" or STAT item.

If the nurse obtains the item, the nurse is responsible for handling the charge tag and recording it on the control/anticipation sheet.

This notation will help control lost charges. If both the item and the charge tag disappear but the item was noted on the control/anticipation sheet, the charge can still be processed accurately.

This is especially true if a nurse "borrows" an item from one Nurserver and puts it into another.

When the chargeable item is actually used for or by the patient, the charge tag is removed and placed on the control/anticipation sheet in the Nurserver.

*A credit is placed when the item charged to the patient is not used or is contaminated or destroyed by the nurse or physician.

Affected Departments

Reviewed _____

PATIENT CHARGE
CONTROL/ANTICIPATION SHEET

DATE _____

SUPPLY TECHNICIAN _____

Imprinting Zone

CHARGEABLE TAGS			
			62-00056 Patient Admit Kit

ANTICIPATED SUPPLIES							
QUANTITY	ITEM	ORDERED BY	FILLED BY	QUANTITY	ITEM	ORDERED BY	FILLED BY

Subject	Effective Date 1-90	Latest Revision & Date
ORDERING EXTRA SUPPLIES		

The nurse anticipates the supplies needed for each patient for the next 24 hours. The 24-hour period will be from 3P.M. to 3P.M. Therefore, all anticipated items will be in the Nurserver before 3P.M. on any given day.

1. The nurse enters the items needed for the next 24-hour period on the control/anticipation sheet by writing the description of the item in the "item" column on the appropriate portion of the sheet.

2. The quantities needed are listed in the spaces provided.

3. Initials of the person ordering are placed in the space provided.

4. At 2P.M. the supply technician begins to fill anticipated items.

5. The supply technician then enters the quantity filled in the appropriate column on the control/anticipation sheet.

6. The supply technician places his or her initials in the space provided.

7. The items are placed in the Nurserver.

8. Items not in stock in the patient care unit are obtained from dispatch.

9. When the specially ordered items arrive from dispatch, the supply technician places the items in the Nurserver, following the proper procedure (see steps 5 and 6 above).

10. The full control/anticipation sheet is reconciled and replaced with a new one every other day or at patient discharge or transfer.

11. If a nurse wishes to have any extra items removed, she or he simply draws a line through the items and the quantity ordered.

Affected Departments

Reviewed _____

Subject	Effective Date	Latest Revision & Date
"CALLED FOR" ITEMS	1-90	

"Called for" items are any extra supplies needed <u>before</u> the scheduled time, i.e., that cannot wait until the next delivery.

1. If the item is needed as soon as possible (ASAP) (within one hour), the nurse requests the item through the administrative communications clerk (ACC). The supply technician brings the item and then writes the description, quantity ordered, and quantity filled on the control/anticipation sheet.

2. If the item is <u>not</u> needed within an hour, the nurse or clerk enters the description and quantity on the control/ anticipation sheet in the appropriate columns. When a nurse has ordered the item on the sheet, she or he then calls the ACC and communicates the order. The ACC contacts the supply technician. If the ACC has ordered the item, he or she contacts the supply technician directly. The supply technician enters the quantity filled when he or she places the supply in the Nurserver.

3. Items required between one and 24 hours should be ordered in the same manner as those needed in 24 hours, since the nurse must anticipate these supplies every 24 hours.

Affected Departments

Reviewed _____

Page 1 of 2

Subject		Effective Date 1-90	Latest Revision & Date
"CALLED FOR FOR" ITEMS (cont.)			

DISPATCH SCHEDULE

Time	Cart	Quantity	From (Area, Floor)	To (Area, Floor)	Cart Lift
7A.M.	Breakfast	12	Dietary	Galley (2, 3, 4)	#1
7:15A.M.	Linen	13	Dispatch	Clean hold (2, 3, 4)	#1
8:30A.M.	Empty linen carts returned		Clean hold (2, 3, 4)	Dispatch	#1
9A.M.	Return dietary carts		Soiled hold (2, 3, 4)	Decontamination	#2
9:30A.M.	Clean dietary and trash carts		Dietary	Galley (2, 3, 4)	#1
10:45A.M.	Dietary lunch carts		Dietary	Galley (2, 3, 4)	#1
1P.M.	Return lunch carts		Soiled hold (2, 3, 4)	Decontamination	#2
1:30P.M.	Supply carts		Clean hold (2, 3, 4)	Dispatch	#1
1:30P.M.	Pharmacy carts		Pharmacy	Clean hold (2, 3, 4)	#1

Work performed by the fourth floor supply technician during the week; second floor supply technician on weekends:

On call	Supply carts		Dispatch	Emergency room physical therapy, recovery, and cardiac catheterization laboratory	#1
2—3:30P.M.	Fill anticipatory orders		Dispatch	2, 3, 4	
10A.M.—4P.M.	Housekeeping will pick up trash and soiled linen				
7:15A.M., 10A.M., 1P.M., and 3P.M.	Specimen to laboratory		Soiled hold	Laboratory	Carry by hand

Affected Departments

Reviewed _____

Subject	Effective Date 1-90	Latest Revision & Date
STAT ORDERS		

1. A STAT order is for <u>emergencies only</u> and should be designated as such. These are generally medical supply items. When a STAT order is received by the ACC, he or she immediately alerts the supply technician by voice or beeper. The supply technician stops whatever he or she is doing and obtains the item by the quickest means possible.

2. The supply technician delivers the item to the nurse who ordered it.

3. If the person who ordered the item is not available (i.e., not in room, etc.), the supply technician contacts someone on the medical team (another nurse or ACC) to let him or her know the item has been delivered.

4. After giving the item to the nursing personnel, the supply technician records all items delivered on the control/anticipation sheet in that Nurserver.

5. The supply technician is available for any follow-up STAT orders, especially in critical situations.

6. If the nurse contacts the supply technician directly, the same procedure (see steps 1 through 5) is followed.

7. When the supply technician is not on duty, STAT calls are placed by telephone or intercom directly to the dispatch office. The dispatcher will obtain the items and send them to their destinations either through the pneumatic tube, cart lift, or the service elevator.

Affected Departments

Reviewed _____

Page 1 of 1

Subject	Effective Date	Latest Revision & Date
PROCEDURAL INSTRUMENT TRAYS	1-90	

1. Procedural trays are issued <u>only</u> after being ordered on the control/anticipation sheet by the ACC.

2. When the order has been received, the tray requested is obtained from the supply room or from dispatch.

3. The tray is taken to the Nurserver, entered on the control/anticipation sheet, and placed on the proper shelf.

4. If the tray is generally "stocked" on the floor, dispatch is advised so that a replacement can be issued to restock the quantity kept on that floor.

5. When the tray has been used, it is returned to decontamination via the soiled cart lift.

6. Any discrepancies or losses must be reported immediately to the materials management manager and to nursing.

7. All trays and sterile items must be checked daily for expiration dates.

8. If a tray is unavailable on a particular floor and is needed for use, dispatch is called.

9. If it is unavailable from dispatch, a tray is obtained from another floor and dispatch is informed so a replacement can be sent there.

Affected Departments

Reviewed _____

Subject	Effective Date	Latest Revision & Date
RENTAL EQUIPMENT	1-90	

1. Follow Procedure #8.10 (see steps 1 to 4).

2. When the item has been discounted, the charge must be processed accordingly. Dispatch coordinates the control of equipment with assistance from the supply technician.

   a. The supply technician visually verifies that equipment is in the patient room and sends a list daily to dispatch for review with control board and suspense file.

   b. Dispatch notifies the supply technician if equipment is missing, for follow-up.

Affected Departments

Reviewed _____

Page 1 of 1

Subject	Effective Date	Latest Revision & Date
ORTHOPEDIC EQUIPMENT	1-90	

1. The ACC notifies the supply technician of requests for traction equipment.

2. The supply technician obtains the necessary equipment from dispatch.

3. After the equipment has been placed in the patient's room, the supply technician takes the equipment charge ticket and files it in the equipment file.

4. When equipment is removed from the patient's room, the supply technician processes the charge.

5. During the evening and night shifts, when a supply technician is not on duty, the nurse or ACC contacts the dispatcher. The dispatcher sends the item to the floor (if it is not already on the "fracture cart" stored on the orthopedic floor). The nurse is responsible for setting up or dismantling the traction equipment.

Affected Departments

Reviewed _____

Subject	Effective Date	Latest Revision & Date
CODE BLUE	1-90	

1. If a Code Blue is called, the supply technician in the area of the code (same zone or floor) stops all other duties and returns to the clean hold room to be available for supply or equipment orders.

2. If two supply technicians are on duty, one remains in the clean hold room to handle orders, and one stays on the zone, as scheduled.

3. The supply technician must stay out of the way of the team responding to the code.

4. The supply technician provides only what is requested.

Affected Departments

Reviewed _____

Page 1 of 1

Subject	Effective Date	Latest Revision & Date
FLOOR STOCK TRAYS/EQUIPMENT	1-90	

1 Crash cart
1 IV cutdown tray
1 Suture pack
2 Chest tubes
   Thoracic catheters:
   1 36 French
   1 28 French
1 Underwater drainage set
1 Tracheotomy tray
3 Clot evacuators (on the surgical floor)
1 Arterial blood sampling kit
1 Subclavian tray
1 Venisection tray
2 Oral suction machines
1 Gastric suction machine
1 CVP tray

(See Procedure #8.10 for obtaining and replacing these and other trays and equipment.)

Affected Departments

Reviewed _____

Subject		Effective Date	Latest Revision & Date
DISCHARGES AND TRANSFERS		1-90	

When a patient is <u>discharged</u>, all supply charges must be processed <u>that day</u>. Any credits should also be processed.

When a patient is <u>transferred</u> to another room, all charges should be reconciled and processed the same day.

Nursing notifies the supply technician or dispatcher when a transfer or discharge is to take place. As much advance notice as possible should be given.

The supply technician counts supplies in the Nurserver, processes the charges, and restocks the Nurserver for use by the next patient. Extra items and equipment are removed from the Nurserver and returned to materials management. A new control/anticipation sheet is placed in the Nurserver.

The patient's personal property is the responsibility of nursing personnel.

Affected Departments

Reviewed _____

Page 1 of 1

Subject	Effective Date 1-90	Latest Revision & Date
ROUTINE SPECIMEN HANDLING/TRANSPORT		

Specimens collected by nursing personnel are placed in a clean, leak-proof container with a securely fastened lid.

The specimen is taken by nursing to the refrigerator located in the soiled hold room on that floor.

If any spillage or leakage occurs, nursing takes care of the cleanup or transfer of the specimen to another container.

Specimens are routinely routed to the laboratory at 7:30A.M., 10A.M., 1:30P.M., 4P.M., 7P.M., and 10P.M.

Routine specimen transport from 7A.M. to 3:30P.M. is the responsibility of the supply technician. Departments on the first floor will deliver specimens themselves.

After 3:30P.M., nursing and laboratory personnel assume the responsibility for coordinating specimen handling. Laboratory personnel do the transporting.

Specimens are taken from the refrigerator and placed in a plastic tub/tote box. The tote box is closed (lid attached) and is placed on a miscellaneous cart.

The cart is moved to the cart lift in the clean hold room and placed into position, and the lift's send button is pushed.

The cart lift automatically transports the cart to the dispatch area (on the lower level).

The dispatcher consolidates the tote boxes from all three floors onto one cart and sends the cart to the first floor clean hold room.

The dispatcher calls the laboratory to announce that the cart is on the way.

Laboratory personnel pick up the specimens in the clean hold room and return the cart and tote boxes to dispatch.

Dispatch sends the cart and tote boxes back to their assigned locations.

For handling of STAT specimens, see Procedure #8.17.

Affected Departments

Reviewed _____

Page 1 of 1

Subject	Effective Date 1-90	Latest Revision & Date
STAT SPECIMEN HANDLING		

All STAT specimens are processed by laboratory personnel.

The ACC notifies the laboratory when a STAT specimen needs processing.

Affected Departments

Reviewed _____

Subject	Effective Date	Latest Revision & Date
CLEANING NURSERVERS	1-90	

The Nurservers are completely emptied and fully cleaned once a month, starting the first full week of the month. In-between cleanup is done as needed.

Housekeeping cleans the Nurservers (supply section only). Starting with the lowest numbered rooms, four Nurservers are cleaned each day, five days a week, on each zone.

The supply technician empties the Nurserver first thing in the morning (7 A.M.) and notifies the housekeeping personnel working in that zone.

When the Nurserver is completely cleaned, the housekeeping personnel leave a tent card on the shelf, and the supply technician returns all supplies to the Nurserver. Each day, the cleaning progresses to the next four Nurservers (e.g., Monday: rooms 201, 202, 203, 204; Tuesday: rooms 205, 206, 207, 208; Wednesday: rooms 209, 210, 211, 212; and so on in each zone).

Affected Departments

Reviewed _____

SECTION IX

DISPATCHING
SECTION IX

Subject	Effective Date 1-90	Latest Revision & Date
DISPATCHING OVERVIEW		

Dispatch functions as the control and communications center for materials management.

Dispatch's primary responsibilities are: delivery of supplies and equipment, patient charge systems, STAT order processing, night medications, the pneumatic tube system (PTS), the cart lifts, the linen/trash tube system, and patient care mobile equipment management.

The dispatch office is staffed 24 hours a day, 7 days a week.

If other areas of materials management are closed, the dispatcher covers and handles all situations.

Affected Departments

Reviewed _____

Page 1 of 1

Subject	Effective Date 1-90	Latest Revision & Date
DISPATCH CENTER		

The dispatch center is that area of materials management that contains patient care supply items in ready-to-use condition.

The types of items kept in this area are:

1. Disposable sterile and nonsterile medical supplies (chargeable and nonchargeable)
2. Reusable sterile supplies (floor instrument trays)
3. Rental equipment (orthopedic, suction, thermia units, etc.)
4. Inventory items
5. Noninventory (direct purchase) items
6. Pharmacy night medications

The dispatch center is a clean area. All items stored there are used for direct patient care. Items are stored on wire racks/carts to provide flexibility, accessibility, and a clean environment.

Chargeable supply items are stored on the shelves with the appropriate charge tag attached to each item.

Inventory items are primarily obtained from the storeroom. A back-up stock is maintained in the dispatch center. Item locations are found in the locator file kept in the dispatch office.

Inventory items issued from dispatch must be so documented on a stock requisition.

Items issued that are noninventory (direct purchase) are charged to the user department in the interdepartmental supply transfer book. Direct purchase items stored in this area are inventoried and reordered, when necessary, by the dispatcher, through the purchasing department.

Items issued that are patient chargeable are sent with the appropriate charge tag attached to each item.

Affected Departments

Reviewed _____

Subject	Effective Date	Latest Revision & Date
STERILE STORES	1-90	

Sterile stores contains all items used to support the case cart system for surgery, delivery, and the outpatient surgery and treatment functions.

This includes:

1. Sterile surgical packs
2. Sterile surgical instrument sets
3. Sterile disposable surgical supplies
4. Sterile surgical tools and utensils

All items stored in this area are sterile and in ready-to-use condition.

All items in this area come from three sources:

1. Inventory
2. Processing
3. Direct purchase

All inventory items placed in this area are charged to the user department when issued. Items returned unused need a credit document.

All items from processing are placed on shelves in their designated location on a quota basis. The shelves are restocked daily by processing personnel and are rotated to avoid outdated supplies.

Direct purchase items are ordered through the purchasing department by processing personnel and are charged to the user department as issued.

Affected Departments

Reviewed _____

Page 1 of 1

Subject		Effective Date 1-90	Latest Revision & Date
	CART LIFT SYSTEM		

All supply carts are to be transported to user departments via the cart lift. Transport of carts both to and from materials management is the responsibility of and must be coordinated through the dispatch office. Carts are delivered and returned based on a predetermined schedule. Random cart activity also requires coordination.

The cart lift system is designed to semiautomatically load, transport, and unload (eject) carts that have an adapting device (coupler) for the system. Other carts of proper size can be transported via the cart lift (carts measuring $24^5/_8$ inches wide × 52 inches long × $49^1/_2$ inches high).

Maintenance of cart lifts is provided by the manufacturer's representative or the institution's maintenance personnel. Whenever a breakdown occurs, the maintenance department is notified immediately; its personnel make necessary repairs or contact the manufacturer for service.

Affected Departments

Reviewed _____

Page 1 of 1

Subject		Effective Date	Latest Revision & Date
	CART LIFT BREAKDOWN	1-90	

If any of the cart lifts break down, all affected departments are immediately notified (the ACC on patient floors and surgery), and maintenance is contacted. The materials management manager in charge should also be notified.

If repairs can be made in a short time so that patient care will not be jeopardized, the transport of carts is delayed until repairs are made.

Before repairs are made, either the other operational modes of the cart lift are used to transport scheduled carts, or the staff elevators are used. In that case, dispatch personnel or supply technicians accompany carts to their destination (floor only).

Affected Departments

Reviewed _____

Page 1 of 1

Subject	Effective Date 1-90	Latest Revision & Date
OPERATING THE PNEUMATIC TUBE SYSTEM (PTS)		

The PTS connects 23 different stations (departments) throughout the institution with an automated means of transporting small supply items and paperwork/mail. (Items must be smaller than 6 inches × 15 inches to fit inside the cylindrically shaped carrier.)

The PTS is monitored and controlled by a small computer located in the dispatch office.

The PTS uses impact-resistant plastic carriers or "tubes" to hold the items that are being transported. These carriers travel through a network of tubes by forced air pressure or vacuum at a high rate of speed, arriving at any destination (station) in less than 30 seconds.

Each station is assigned a number of carriers to handle its volume of activity. These are reallocated or updated periodically or whenever necessary.

Operating the PTS

A carrier is loaded with the items to be transported. It must be closed tightly. If a carrier opens during transit, it will jam the system.

A completed routing slip (see sample) must be included in case the carrier is sent to the wrong place. It can then be forwarded to the desired destination.

The carrier is closed and placed in the "send" slot at the station.

The code number for the desired destination is found on the control/director panel. Pushing the proper buttons on the "keyboard" will enter this number.

At this point the computer takes over, directs the carrier through the system, and deposits the carrier at its destination.

At the receiving station, the carrier is removed from the "receive slot," opened, emptied of the contents, and placed back in the storage slot.

The transaction is completed.

Affected Departments

Reviewed _____

Subject	Effective Date	Latest Revision & Date
OPERATING THE PNEUMATIC TUBE SYSTEM (PTS) (con't.)	1-90	

If the storage slot at the receiving station is full, the destination's station is unavailable. The carrier will not leave, and the computer will know not to send it.

In this case:

1. The receiving department can be called by telephone to be notified that its station is unavailable so that it can be cleared.
2. The carrier can be sent to the next closest station.
3. An item can be hand-carried to its destination.
4. The delivery can be postponed to the next day.

If system malfunction occurs, the maintenance department is contacted immediately.

PTS ROUTING SLIP

DATE _____

SENT FROM _____

SENT TO _____

Affected Departments

Reviewed _____

Subject	Effective Date	Latest Revision & Date
TRASH/LINEN TUBE SYSTEM	1-90	

The trash/linen tube system automatically transports soiled linen and trash through a 20-inch-diameter tube from each station to the dock area, where trash is compacted and linen is held in a separate room for pickup by the commercial laundry.

A separate tube transports soiled linen, and another transports trash. The tubes are powered by a large motor that creates suction to draw the material through the system.

The tubes are routed away from all other traffic paths to keep soiled material away from patients, staff, and visitors. In addition, the use of the tubes eliminates handling by in-house personnel and reduces traffic on elevators.

A station for the trash tube and the linen tube is located in the soiled utility room on each floor of the facility.

The tube will accept only an 18-inch bag of material. Other sizes will jam the system. Bags should not be overstuffed.

<u>Operating the trash and linen tubes</u>

The bagged linen and trash are taken to the tube station.

Linen is placed in the GREEN tube station; trash is placed in the RED tube station.

No more than three (3) bags are put in the station bin at one time.

The door is closed tightly. The operating <u>button</u> is pushed, and the bags are transported through the system to their destinations.

If the door is held open and bags are thrown in continuously, the system will jam.

If a bag breaks while being loaded into the bin, the suction of the system will carry all the contents through the tubes.

If the system does not take the bags away, another station is being used at the same time. The system will not allow more than one station to be used at the same time. If no results are obtained after a few minutes, maintenance should be contacted.

If any malfunction occurs, maintenance should be contacted immediately.

Affected Departments

Reviewed _____

Subject		Effective Date 1-90	Latest Revision & Date
DISPATCH SCHEDULE			

Time	Cart	Quantity	From (Area, Floor)	To (Area, Floor)	Cart Lift
6:45 A.M.	Breakfast	12	Kitchen (LL)	Galley (2, 3, 4)	#1
7:30 A.M.	Specimen	3	Clean hold (2, 3, 4)	Laboratory (1)	#1
8 A.M.	Trash/ miscellaneous	4	Dispatch (LL)	Clean hold (1, 2, 3, 4)	#1
8:10 A.M.	Supply and linen	16	Dispatch (LL)	Physical therapy, radiology, emergency, recovery, cardiac catheterization laboratory (1)	#1
8:30 A.M.	Supply and linen	16	Physical therapy, radiology, emergency, recovery, cardiac catheterization laboratory (1)	Dispatch (LL)	#1
8:50 A.M.	Breakfast	12	Galley (2, 3, 4)	Decontamination (LL)	#2
9:15 A.M.	Nourishments	3	Kitchen/dispatch (LL)	Galley (2, 3, 4)	#1
9:45 A.M.	Nourishments	3	Galley (2, 3, 4)	Dispatch/kitchen (LL)	#1
10 A.M.	Specimen	3	Clean hold (2, 3, 4)	Laboratory (1)	#1
10:45 A.M.	Lunch	12	Kitchen/dispatch (LL)	Galley (2, 3, 4)	#1
11:45 A.M.	Linen	14	Dispatch (LL)	Clean hold (2, 3, 4)	#1
12 NOON	Linen	14	Clean hold (2, 3, 4)	Dispatch (LL)	#1
12:15 P.M.	Lunch	12	Galley (2, 3, 4)	Decontamination (LL)	#2
1 P.M.	Specimen	3	Clean hold (2, 3, 4)	Laboratory (1)	#1
1:15 P.M.	Trash/ miscellaneous	4	Dispatch (LL)	Clean hold (2, 3, 4)	#1
1:30 P.M.	Unit dose	3	Pharmacy/dispatch (LL)	Clean hold (2, 3, 4)	#1
2 P.M.	Nourishments	3	Kitchen/dispatch (LL)	Galley (2, 3, 4)	#1

Affected Departments

Reviewed _____

Subject	Effective Date	Latest Revision & Date
DISPATCH SCHEDULE (cont.)	1-90	

Time	Cart	Quantity	From (Area, Floor)	To (Area, Floor)	Cart Lift
2:30P.M.	Unit dose	3	Clean hold (2, 3, 4)	Dispatch/pharmacy (LL)	#1
2:35P.M.	Nourishments	3	Galley (2, 3, 4)	Dispatch/kitchen (LL)	#1
2:45P.M.	Supply	10	Dispatch (LL)	Clean hold (2, 3, 4)	#1
3P.M.	Supply	10	Clean hold (2, 3, 4)	Dispatch (LL)	#1
4P.M.	Specimen	3	Clean hold (2, 3, 4)	Laboratory (1)	#1
4:30P.M.	Supper	12	Kitchen/dispatch (LL)	Galley (2, 3, 4)	#1
6:15P.M.	Supper	12	Galley (2, 3, 4)	Decontamination (LL)	#2
7P.M.	Specimen	3	Clean hold (2, 3, 4)	Laboratory (1)	#1
10P.M.	Specimen	3	Clean hold (2, 3, 4)	Laboratory (1)	#1
11P.M.	Trash	3	Soiled hold (2, 3, 4)	Decontamination (LL)	#2

Affected Departments

Reviewed _____

Subject	Effective Date 1-90	Latest Revision & Date
SUPPLY REQUISITION		

The dispatch office receives calls for a variety of items and handles a variety of activities.

All transactions handled by the dispatch office are so noted on the supply requisition. (See sample.)

The supply requisitions are periodically reviewed by the distribution manager to evaluate the volume and type of activity.

SUPPLY REQUISITION

DATE _____   DEPARTMENT _____

COST CENTER # _____   ROOM # _____

ITEM #	QUANTITY	DISPENSING UNIT	ITEM DESCRIPTION

TIME _____   FILLED BY _____

SENT VIA   PTS ☐   CART LIFT ☐   ELEVATOR ☐

Affected Departments

Reviewed _____

Page 1 of 1

Subject	Effective Date	Latest Revision & Date
REQUESTS FOR SUPPLIES—STAT	1-90	

When patient floor personnel request medical/surgical supplies "STAT," this means that they are needed immediately, i.e., that there is a potential life or death situation.

All STAT calls are handled before all others.

STAT calls are noted on the dispatch log.

Dispatchers will not argue or discuss the validity of a STAT order with the user departments; they will respond first.

STAT calls are not generally accepted for nonmedical items. Requests for such are noted and reported to the manager for follow-up.

Affected Departments

Reviewed _____

Page 1 of 1

Subject	Effective Date 1-90	Latest Revision & Date
LOCATOR FILE		

All items stored in materials management are noted in the locator file.

The locator file, kept in the dispatch office, is a listing of all items with their corresponding location in the department. This is both an alphabetical (by generic name) and numerical (institutional item number) cross-referenced list.

The backup or originating source (storeroom, processing, etc.) is also noted for each item.

The distribution manager reviews the locator file regularly and updates it as necessary. Any changes are made and dated. Notations of changes are highlighted on the department bulletin board.

Affected Departments

Reviewed _____

Subject	Effective Date	Latest Revision & Date
REQUESTS FOR SUPPLIES—STOCK/INVENTORY	1-90	

Departments may request items stored in either the dispatch center or the storeroom.

Inventory items, no matter where they are located, must be charged out, when issued, on a stock requisition form.

Ancillary departments usually order stock items according to the distribution schedule. If they request items from stock, they must present a stock requisition. The dispatch office is authorized to issue supplies from the storeroom or the dispatch center if the order is STAT.

Patient care floors also may request stock items. These floors are not required to fill out a stock requisition. Dispatch office personnel will fill out the stock requisition as the item is issued.

Affected Departments

Reviewed _____

Subject		
REQUEST FOR SUPPLIES—NONSTOCK	Effective Date 1-90	Latest Revision & Date

Departments and patient care floors may request noninventory supply items that are available in the dispatch center.

These items are charged to the department by an interdepartmental supply transfer.

These and all other requests are noted in the dispatch log.

Affected Departments

Reviewed _____

Subject	Effective Date 1-90	Latest Revision & Date
REQUESTS FOR SUPPLIES—PATIENT CHARGEABLE		

All chargeable supplies must have a charge tag attached when issued to patient care floors.

Chargeable supplies are charged out two ways:

1. Inventory (stock) items are charged from stock and then sent to the floor.

2. Noninventory items are sent to the user. They have already been charged to materials management.

Affected Departments

Reviewed _____

Page 1 of 1

Subject REQUESTS FOR SUPPLIES—INTERDEPARTMENTAL TRANSFERS	Effective Date 1-90	Latest Revision & Date

Departments may request supplies that are noninventory items, purchased directly by materials management and stored in the dispatch center.

These items are charged out, when requested, via an interdepartmental supply transfer. (See sample.) Materials management fills out the transfer form for nursing areas. Ancillary departments fill out their own.

When filling out the transfer, the following should be noted:

1. Date
2. Department issued to (cost center number)
3. Item
4. Quantity
5. Cost

Interdepartmental supply transfers are totaled and forwarded to accounting for actual transfer to the user department's budget.

Affected Departments

Reviewed _____

Procedure #9.15

<u>INTERDEPARTMENTAL SUPPLY</u>
<u>TRANSFER</u>

DATE _____

TRANSFER FROM: DEPARTMENT_____ COST CENTER#_____

TRANSFER TO: DEPARTMENT_____ COST CENTER #_____

QUANTITY		CODE	DESCRIPTION	UNIT	UNIT/ COST	TOTAL
REQ'D	TRANS					

TOTAL QUANTITY DELIVERED				TOTAL COST	
REQUESTED BY			APPROVED BY		

ORIGINAL — TRANSFER FROM DEPARTMENT

Copy 1 — Data Processing

278

Subject	Effective Date	Latest Revision & Date
REQUEST FOR NIGHT MEDICATIONS	1-90	

The dispatch office handles distribution of medications when the pharmacy is closed (11P.M. to 7A.M., Monday through Friday).

Night medications are stored in the night medications cabinet in the dispatch center in <u>numbered sequence</u>.

Patient floors requesting medications call the dispatch office and request the medication <u>BY NUMBER ONLY</u>.

The dispatcher obtains the requested medications from the cabinet and signs them out on the night medications control sheet. (See sample.) In addition, the request is noted on the dispatch log.

Narcotics are not stored in the night medications cabinet. They are available in the team conference center on each patient zone.

The pharmacy inventories the night medications cabinet and restocks it each day at 9A.M. Any discrepancies are reviewed immediately with the director of materials management and the dispatch staff.

Affected Departments

Reviewed _____

Page 1 of 1

NIGHT MEDICATIONS
CONTROL SHEET

DATE/TIME	DEPARTMENT REQUESTING	ITEM #	QUANTITY	ISSUED BY	RESTOCKED BY	DATE

Subject	Effective Date	Latest Revision & Date
REQUESTS FOR EQUIPMENT	1-90	

Rental equipment is requested for the patient care floors via the appropriate requisition filled out with:

1. Patient name
2. Identification number
3. Room number
4. Date
5. Item/quantity requested

The requisition may be transmitted by nursing personnel or the supply technicians.

The dispatcher obtains the item and transports it to the destination via the quickest, most direct means:

1. PTS (if item is small enough; 6 inches × 15 inches)
2. Cart lift (if item will fit into convertible cart and onto lift)
3. Staff elevator (if taken up elevator, items must be accompanied by the dispatcher and taken to the floor's clean hold room; dispatch personnel do not take the items to the patient's room)

For proper handling of the charges and equipment control, refer to Procedure #9.18.

Affected Departments

Reviewed _____

Page 1 of 1

Subject	Effective Date	Latest Revision & Date
EQUIPMENT CONTROL	1-90	

All rental equipment is rotated and controlled by a locator or equipment control board. Each piece of equipment is numbered. When a piece of equipment is ordered, the dispatcher determines which unit is sent by moving the tag of that item on the control board and putting it on the hook corresponding to the patient room number to which it is to be sent.

The tag is removed from the room number hook when the item is returned from processing and placed behind the rest of the tags for that type of item.

When a piece of equipment is taken to maintenance or sent in for repair, the corresponding tag of that item is removed from the board and placed on the "repair" hook.

When an item is issued, an entry is made for the equipment and held in a "suspense" file by dispatch until it is discontinued or returned to processing.

The patient discharge report is reviewed daily by the dispatcher. If the patient has been charged and the equipment not yet returned, dispatch calls the supply technician to verify that item's status and location.

The dispatcher then transfers the status from the suspense file to the patient-charging file.

If the patient is transferred to another room, the charge is changed and the tag on the equipment control board is moved to the appropriate room number hook.

If the dispatcher or supply technician finds that patient care personnel change the location of the equipment without having the item cleaned or inspected by materials management, the incidents will be reviewed with the patient care staff and manager and then documented and presented to the distribution manager or director of materials management for follow-up.

Affected Departments

Reviewed _____

Page 1 of 1

Subject	Effective Date	Latest Revision & Date
SUPPLY RETURNS/EXCHANGES	1-90	

Departments wishing to return or exchange supplies with materials management must present the __unused__ items to the dispatch office with a completed stock requisition (if stock items) or interdepartmental supply transfer (if nonstock items).

Materials management does not accept returns of used or semiused items, nor items that are being discarded by departments because they are obsolete. These types of items should be discussed with the distribution manager for proper disposition.

Affected Departments

Reviewed _____

Page 1 of 1

Subject	Effective Date	Latest Revision & Date
HANDLING EMERGENCY, EARLY, OR LATE DELIVERIES	1-90	

The dispatch office handles incoming items at the receiving dock when receiving personnel are not available or during off-duty hours. This includes: pharmacy, dietary, linen, blood, flowers, and other items that may arrive.

Delivery personnel will push a doorbell to notify dispatch that they have arrived. The bell rings in the dispatch center.

The dispatcher notifies security when someone arrives at the dock after hours, so that security personnel can accompany dispatch staff to the dock for safety reasons.

For proper handling and dissemination, refer to receiving (stock and direct items) procedures.

Affected Departments

Reviewed _____

Subject	Effective Date 1-90	Latest Revision & Date
REQUESTS FOR EMERGENCY CASE CARTS		

The dispatch office, staffed 24 hours a day, 7 days a week, may be called on to set up an emergency case cart for use in surgery or delivery.

Surgery will call materials management and verbally request the emergency case cart. This cart is set up at all times and is on standby in the sterile stores area to be used only for emergencies.

The emergency case cart contains basic instruments, supplies, and linen packs to begin an emergency case. If other instrument sets or packs are required, surgery states this during its telephone request.

Materials management personnel treat this request as top priority, stock the case cart, and send it immediately via the cart lift.

If the appropriate case cart requisition cannot be sent when the telephone call is made, surgery will send it as soon as possible so that cart setup and use is documented, and so that another emergency cart can be set up for subsequent emergencies. The second emergency cart is stocked immediately following verification that the first cart has been used.

Affected Departments

Reviewed _____

Page 1 of 1

Subject	Effective Date 1-90	Latest Revision & Date
EMERGENCY SUPPLIES		

The dispatch office, open 24 hours a day, 7 days a week, is responsible for obtaining supplies that are needed when the purchasing office is closed.

If supplies cannot be found anywhere in the institution, the dispatcher acts as the materials management department representative and obtains the items needed from whatever source possible: vendor, other healthcare facility, local supply mart, etc.

Affected Departments

Reviewed _____

Page 1 of 1

Subject	Effective Date	Latest Revision & Date
NOURISHMENTS AND LATE TRAYS	1-90	

Nourishment carts and "hold" or late trays are sent to all patient floors daily at 9:30A.M. and 2:30P.M.

Dietary prepares the carts and delivers them to the dispatch area.

Dispatch sends them to the floors via the cart lift.

The supply technician takes the carts to the respective galley.

Dietary personnel put all nourishments away and return the carts to the clean hold room for return to the lower level and, then, to the kitchen.

Affected Departments

Reviewed _____

Page 1 of 1

Subject	Effective Date 1-90	Latest Revision & Date
ORTHOPEDIC TRACTION CART		

The orthopedic traction cart is stocked daily (as needed) by the supply technician assigned to the orthopedic area.

The "fracture cart" is stocked and remains in the dispatch area on standby status. The cart is ordered by the supply technician or the ACC and sent up via the staff elevator by the dispatcher.

After use, the cart is returned to dispatch, where it is restocked and checked to see that all patient charges have been processed.

Affected Departments

Reviewed _____

Page 1 of 1

Subject		Effective Date 1-90	Latest Revision & Date
EQUIPMENT RECORDS			

Materials management maintains records of repairs and maintenance performed on all equipment items.

The equipment maintenance record form (see sample) is completed for each piece of equipment in the department and is updated whenever maintenance is performed.

Affected Departments

Reviewed _____

EQUIPMENT MAINTENANCE RECORD

ITEM _____ ID # _____ MANUFACTURER _____

VENDOR _____ MODEL _____ SERIAL # _____ COST _____

DATE PLACED IN SERVICE _____ PURCHASE ORDER # _____ DEPARTMENT/LOCATION _____

WARRANTY EXPIRES _____ INSPECTION FREQUENCY _____ SERVICED BY _____

PREVENTIVE MAINTENANCE REQUIREMENTS _____

_____

_____

REMARKS _____

_____

EQUIPMENT SERVICE

DATE OUT OF SERVICE	DATE SENT	FACTORS CHECKED ACCORDING TO MANUFACTURER'S REQUIREMENTS/INSTRUCTIONS	REPAIRS RENDERED	REPAIRED BY	DATE EQUIPMENT INSPECTED	INSPECTED BY	DATE RETURNED TO DEPARTMENT

Subject	Effective Date	Latest Revision & Date
PATIENT TRANSPORT REQUESTS	1-90	

See Section XV.

Affected Departments

Reviewed _____

Subject	Effective Date	Latest Revision & Date
CARDIAC CATHETERIZATION LABORATORY SUPPLIES AND EQUIPMENT	1-90	

<u>Supplies:</u>

All supplies for the catheterization laboratory are stored on and transported via a supply cart.

Materials management stocks the cart and dispatches it via the clean cart lift to the first-floor clean hold room at 6A.M., <u>Monday through Friday</u>, where laboratory personnel pick it up and transport it to the catheterization laboratory. The cart is returned to materials management by the catheterization laboratory personnel at the end of the procedure(s) that same day.

<u>Nonstock catheters</u> and backup supplies are stored on a cart in the cardiac diagnostics area. These supplies are monitored by catheterization laboratory personnel and ordered via a traveling requisition card or nonstock request for purchasing services form through the purchasing office.

On arrival, these supplies are delivered directly to the catheterization laboratory for acceptance.

<u>Reprocessed supplies and equipment:</u>

After a catheterization procedure, catheterization laboratory personnel transport items to be reprocessed to the soiled hold room (first floor), place them in a gray tote box, and put them on a cart to be sent to materials management/decontamination immediately.

Materials management reprocesses all instruments, transducers, and equipment according to the proper sterilizing technique and has the items ready for the next day's scheduled cases by 6A.M.

These processed items are returned to the catheterization laboratory via the supply cart, sent daily at 6A.M.

<u>Emergency supply needs:</u>

When the catheterization laboratory plans to do more than two (2) procedures on a given day, it notifies materials management. Items stored in materials management that are needed for the procedures are dispatched to the clean hold room as soon after notification as possible.

Other instruments, transducers, and equipment to be used are obtained from the backup cart in cardiac diagnostics by catheterization laboratory personnel.

Affected Departments

Reviewed _____

SECTION X

PATIENT SUPPLY CHARGE SYSTEM
SECTION X

Subject	Effective Date 1-90	Latest Revision & Date
PATIENT SUPPLY CHARGE SYSTEM OVERVIEW		

The healthcare institution earns revenue by charging for the resources used in patient care.

The resources used may be supply items, equipment, and instruments.

The criteria for determining whether an item is directly charged to individual patients includes:

1. Value/cost of $10 or more
2. Acceptability to the marketplace: preferred provider organizations (PPOs), commercial insurance, employers, or patients.
3. Volume of items used annually
4. Uniqueness to patient treatment

Chargeable supplies are then "sold" to the patient at a "price" that exceeds the hospital's cost by a reasonable markup/profit. The "sale" transaction occurs through the patient accounting/billing system.

The costs and revenues for chargeable supplies are allocated to the user department, since the user is closest to the actual activity/transaction and can better control the capturing of the charges.

Affected Departments

Reviewed _____

Page 1 of 1

Subject	Effective Date 1-90	Latest Revision & Date
THE CHARGE MASTER		

The charge master lists all patient chargeable items (supply items, equipment, procedural trays, etc.) in both numerical (by item code number) and alphabetical sequence.

The charge master includes the following information:

1. Item number
2. Revenue center code number (department to which the revenue is allocated)
3. Charging unit (each, pack, hour, day, etc.)
4. Unit cost
5. Selling price
6. Item description
7. Inventory number (if different than charge number)

Whenever there is a change in the cost to the hospital, an adjustment in selling price is made accordingly.

The charge master is reprinted quarterly, with all new items added and obsolete items deleted. The charge control clerk is responsible for making sure all corrections, additions, deletions, etc., are made properly.

Affected Departments

Reviewed _____

Subject	Effective Date	Latest Revision & Date
ADDITIONS TO/DELETIONS FROM CHARGE MASTER	1-90	

Patient chargeable supplies are generally considered to be those that will have a <u>unit cost</u> of $10 or more.

When a new supply is purchased that will become patient chargeable, the charge master is updated.

This notification form is sent to data processing after it has been verified that the item is not in inventory (to avoid a duplicate item being assigned two [2] code numbers).

Data processing will assign the code number and return a copy of the notification form to the requesting department. The code number is then ready for use.

The requesting department will also receive an updated charge master showing the item added to the file.

The description and price should be verified. Any errors should be immediately corrected.

Affected Departments

Reviewed _____

Page 1 of 1

Subject	Effective Date	Latest Revision & Date
ESTABLISHING PATIENT SUPPLY/EQUIPMENT CHARGES	1-90	

Charges for supplies and equipment are determined by analyzing all costs associated with the procurement and use of the item.

When the total per-use cost of the item has been determined (see sample work sheet), it is then "marked up" according to a predetermined formula (see below). That "selling price" is entered into the charge master, and this remains the price until the cost increases or decreases.

Annually, or as necessary, finance and materials management personnel review the method used to define costs and the subsequent "markup" formula and compare it with the marketplace, third-party payor contracts, etc.

The markup formula is as follows:

Unit cost	Markup factor
$ 10-20	1.20
$ 20-50	1.30
$ 50-100	1.35
$100-500	1.20
$500 or more	1.15

Affected Departments

Reviewed _____

Subject	Effective Date	Latest Revision & Date
ESTABLISHING PATIENT SUPPLY/EQUIPMENT CHARGES (cont.)	1-90	

<u>COST/PRICE WORK SHEET</u>

DEPARTMENT NAME _____ DATE _____

ITEM NAME _____

ITEM USE _____

ESTIMATED ANNUAL USAGE _____ CHARGE CODE # _____

<u>REUSABLE ITEMS' COSTS:</u> (add attachments when necessary)

<u>A</u> <u>ITEM NAME</u>	<u>B</u> <u>QUANTITY</u>	<u>C</u> <u>UNIT COST</u>	<u>D</u> ESTIMATED LIFETIME (# of expected uses)	<u>E</u> COST PER USE
1)				
2)				
3)				
4)				

TOTAL COST OF REUSABLES (investment) $ _____

TOTAL COST OF REUSABLES APPLIED TO SELLING PRICE
(total of column E) $ _____

<u>DISPOSABLE ITEMS' COSTS:</u> (add attachments when necessary)

<u>A</u> <u>ITEM NAME</u>	<u>B</u> <u>QUANTITY</u>	<u>C</u> <u>UNIT COST</u>	<u>D</u> <u>COST PER USE</u>
1)			
2)			
3)			
4)			
5)			

TOTAL COST OF DISPOSABLES (total of column D) $ _____

TOTAL SUPPLY COSTS (reusable + disposable) $ _____

Affected Departments

Reviewed _____

Subject	Effective Date	Latest Revision & Date
ESTABLISHING PATIENT SUPPLY/EQUIPMENT CHARGES (cont.)	1-90	

COST/PRICE WORK SHEET (cont.)

OVERHEAD COSTS: (add % for heat, lights, administrative costs, etc.)
% APPLIED_____ (multiplied times
total supply costs) $ _____

HANDLING/STORAGE COSTS (0.18 × per-use cost of each
item multiplied times total supply costs) $ _____

TOTAL COST OF OVERHEAD $ _____

TOTAL COSTS (reusables, disposables, overhead) $ _____

LABOR COSTS: (include all steps required to accomplish function: i.e., mix,
              prepare, clean, assemble, inspect, administer, disassemble, etc.)

STEP	MINUTES REQUIRED	LABOR COST PER MINUTE	COST PER STEP

TOTAL LABOR COSTS $ _____

Fringe benefits (% of labor rate) $ _____

TOTAL LABOR COSTS $ _____

TOTAL ALL COSTS $ _____

Multiply times established "markup" percentage   % _____

SELLING PRICE $ _____

EFFECTIVE DATE _____

COMMENTS _____

_____

_____   _____
            (SIGNED)   (DATE)

Affected Departments

Reviewed _____

Subject	Effective Date	Latest Revision & Date
CHARGE TAGS	1-90	

Adhesive tags printed with a description and item code number are used to charge a specific supply item to a specific patient.

Chargeable supply items are sent to the user/patient care areas with charge tags already attached. When the item is used, the tag is removed, placed on the control/anticipation sheet, and ultimately entered into the patient billing system.

The charge control/anticipation sheet (see sample) has the information required to charge the item to the patient properly:

1. Imprinting zone for patient name, identification number, age, date, room number, and name of attending physician

2. Places for several charge tags to be attached when the items are used

3. Preprinted revenue center code number that designates which department will be allocated the revenues

Each day the control/anticipation sheets are processed as follows:

1. Imprinted with the patient's plate (done once each day when a new sheet is set up for each patient)

2. Reconciled by materials management/supply technician

3. Returned to the user department for data entry

Affected Departments

Reviewed _____

Page 1 of 1

PATIENT CHARGE
CONTROL/ANTICIPATION SHEET

DATE _____

SUPPLY TECHNICIAN _____

Imprinting Zone

CHARGEABLE TAGS

			62-00056 Patient Admit Kit

ANTICIPATED SUPPLIES

QUANTITY	ITEM	ORDERED BY	FILLED BY	QUANTITY	ITEM	ORDERED BY	FILLED BY

Subject	Effective Date	Latest Revision & Date
SUPPLY CREDITS	1-90	

A charge tag can be used to <u>credit</u> a patient's account for an incorrectly charged item by writing <u>CREDIT</u> in red ink on the face of the tag and repeating an entry (credit) transaction into the patient billing system.

Affected Departments

Reviewed _____

| Subject | EQUIPMENT RENTALS | Effective Date 1-90 | Latest Revision & Date |

Supply items are usually single-use items and are charged for on a one-time-use basis.

Some patient care equipment is charged for on a rental basis (e.g., orthopedic, suction, heating/cooling units, instrument trays).

To charge a patient for such equipment, a rental equipment charge ticket is used. (See sample.)

When the equipment is issued to the patient, the charge transaction is completed. The number of that piece of equipment is noted on the charge suspense file.

When the equipment returns to materials management, the charge is processed. If the patient's name shows up on the discharge list (checked daily), which shows that the patient cannot be using the equipment any longer, the charge is processed.

If a patient is transferred to another room, which is noted on the daily transfer report, the continued use of equipment must be verified by contacting the patient's floor. After verification, the charge is transferred from the old to the new room number.

At the end of each month and the fiscal year (June 30), all rental charges in the suspense file should be "closed" and processed. A new rental equipment charge should be made for all patients using rental equipment and should be placed in the suspense file until discontinued, or until the fiscal period ends, whichever comes first.

Affected Departments

Reviewed _____

Page 1 of 1

RENTAL EQUIPMENT CHARGE TICKET

SUPPLIES CHARGE TICKET
ELECT. MED. EQUIPMENT #13

Room No.	Location:	Time:

ITEM	CODE	QTY	ITEM	CODE	QTY
ELECT. MED. SUPPLY	78-		ELECT. MED. SUPPLY	78-	
IV Pump	00055		K-Kooler Set-Up	40457	
Oral Suction Aspirator Set-Up	40002		K-Kooler Daily	40473	
Oral Suction Aspirator Daily	40028		K-Thermia Set-Up	40507	
Alternating Pressure Mattress	40051		K-Thermia Daily	40556	
Alternating Pressure Motor Set-Up	40101				
Alternating Pressure Motor Daily	40127		Peri-Light Set-Up	40606	
Alternating Pressure Lapidus Pad (Foam)	40150		Peri-Light Daily	40622	
Alternating Pressure Lap Mach Set-Up	40200		Speed Pak Machine Set-Up	40655	
Alternating Pressure Lap Mach Daily	40226		Speed Pak Machine Daily	40671	
Cir-O-Electric Bed Set-Up	40259		Curity Lamp for Compresses Set-Up	40705	
Cir-O-Electric Bed Daily	40275		Curity Lamp for Compresses Daily	40721	
Emerson Pump Set-Up	40309		Sitz Bath Machines Set-Up	40754	
Emerson Pump Daily	40325		Sitz Bath Machines Daily	40770	
Food Pump Set-Up	40358		Sitz Bath Machines Disposable	40804	
Food Pump Daily	40374		Thoracic Pump Gomco Set-Up	40853	
K-Pad Machine Set-Up	40408		Thoracic Pump Gomco Daily	40879	
K-Pad Machine Daily	40424		Stryker Frame Set-Up	40903	

ITEM	CODE	QTY	ITEM	CODE	QTY
ELECT. MED. SUPPLY	78-		ISOLATION	26-	
Stryker Frame Daily	40929		Isolation Set-Up E	00112	
Wangensteen Suc. Gom Levine Set-Up	40952		Isolation Daily	00419	
Wangensteen Suc. Gom Levine Daily	40978		Isolation Set-Up S	00468	
Wangensteen Tray W/Plastic Levine	41000		Isolation Set-Up R	00518	
Wangensteen Tray W/Rubber Levine	41059		Isolation Set-Up P	00567	
Wangensteen Tray W/Salem Sump	41109		Isolation Set-Up W	40050	
Bed Scale Set-Up	41158				
Bed Scale Daily	41174				
K-Thermette Set-Up	40580				
K-Thermette Daily	40598				

305

Subject	Effective Date 1-90	Latest Revision & Date
SPECIAL PATIENT SUPPLY ORDERS		

A patient may require a supply item that is neither routinely stored by the institution nor set up on the patient charge master.

To obtain and charge for such items, the following information is required:

1. All necessary information must be obtained:
   a. Patient's name
   b. Patient's identification number
   c. Room number
   d. Supply item name
   e. Supply item catalog or model number
   f. Quantity required
   g. Cost per item (if available)
   h. Date/time required
   i. Recommended place to purchase item

2. A nonstock request for purchasing services form, including all the above information, is prepared.

3. One copy of the nonstock request for purchasing services form is submitted to purchasing, and one copy is held in the open file.

4. On receipt of the item, a charge tag is prepared with the information required using the miscellaneous charge number (81-00000). The description and selling price (based on the predetermined markup formula) are written on the tag.

5. The item(s) is sent to the patient's floor to be issued to the patient.

6. The copy of the nonstock request for purchasing services form is filed in the closed file.

7. When the item is used, the charge tag is removed for processing according to the routine procedure.

Affected Departments

Reviewed _____

Page 1 of 1

Subject	Effective Date	Latest Revision & Date
MISCELLANEOUS CHARGES	1-90	

Items that are not set up on the charge master and have no charge item code number may be purchased, issued, and charged to patients.

To charge such an item to a patient:

1. A charge tag is obtained and filled out with all the necessary information.

2. The preestablished miscellaneous charge number (81-00000) is used for the item code number in keypunching. It is written in the space provided.

3. The selling price (markup) is established and written in the space provided on the charge tag.

4. The charge tag is attached to the item until used and processed according to the routine procedure.

Affected Departments

Reviewed _____

Subject	Effective Date 1-90	Latest Revision & Date
CHARGE RECONCILIATION		

All patient supply charges must be processed daily to avoid any late charges and ensure timely data entry and billing.

Charges must be reconciled and audited.

Patient charges are reconciled on a sample basis by:

1. Counting 10 percent of chargeable items issued to (placed in) each Nurserver within the last 24 hours. They are written on the control/anticipation sheet. (See sample.) Then, 10 percent of items on each patient care unit supply cart are also sampled/audited.

2. Comparing that count with the number of items or charge tags. A one-for-one match-up must be made; e.g., two bottles of body lotion were put into the Nurserver and noted on the control/anticipation sheet or on the supply cart. At reconciling time, there should be:

   a. Two bottles with charge tags attached, or

   b. Two charge tags on the sheet—and no bottles, or

   c. One bottle with charge tag attached and one charge tag on the sheet

   3. Making out charge tags for any items with tags missing

   4. Pulling charge control/anticipation sheets

   5. Presenting charge control/anticipation sheets to the ACC for imprinting and data entry

Materials management will:

1. Audit several charge control/anticipation sheets and carts, making sure there are tags for all items listed

2. Contact the patient care area manager to make corrections if any discrepancies are found

3. If the reconciliation sample/audit indicates a loss rate of more than the target—6 percent—then all items will be checked/reconciled daily. The process is the same as noted above. If future audits show an acceptable performance, daily reconciliation will not be required.

4. Lost charges are charged to the user departments.

Affected Departments

Reviewed _____

PATIENT CHARGE
CONTROL/ANTICIPATION SHEET

DATE _____

SUPPLY TECHNICIAN _____

Imprinting Zone

CHARGEABLE TAGS

			62-00056 Patient Admit Kit

ANTICIPATED SUPPLIES

QUANTITY	ITEM	ORDERED BY	FILLED BY	QUANTITY	ITEM	ORDERED BY	FILLED BY

Subject	Effective Date 1-90	Latest Revision & Date
LOST CHARGES		

The hospital's financial viability depends on the revenue obtained from patient charges. This includes supply charges.

If a charge is lost (i.e., the charge tag <u>and</u> the item have disappeared), an investigation takes place to determine which patient used the item so that a charge can be made out.

Should the charge tag or the item not be located, the cost (valued at selling price) of that item is charged to the area/department to which the item was distributed.

A lost charge is identified by writing **LOST CHARGE** in the imprinting zone (instead of a specific patient's name and charge number) on the charge control/anticipation sheet and forwarding it to dispatch . All lost charges are totaled and a lost charges report is prepared (see samples).

This procedure is used for lost items of equipment or procedural trays as well as items that are disposable and sterile and were opened but not used, rendering the items unusable. An entry is made on the report for the item, charging it to the department that "lost" it.

The report is submitted to the user department managers for action. If the loss rate is acceptable, daily reconciliation is not required. If not, charges are tracked daily until the rate becomes acceptable.

A summary report of all lost charges is sent to the vice-presidents of finance and nursing at the end of each month. This report includes charges lost because they were processed late (after the patient was discharged).

Affected Departments

Reviewed _____

Procedure #10.11

LOST CHARGES REPORT

DEPARTMENT _____

FOR PERIOD ENDING _____   COST CENTER # _____

DATE	ITEM DESCRIPTION	ITEM CODE #	COST	SELLING PRICE	SUB-TOTAL	TOTAL

Subject	Effective Date	Latest Revision & Date
LATE SUPPLY CHARGES	1-90	

Late charges may occur whenever a patient is discharged and all charge tags have not been processed. The patient's account will remain in audit for two (2) days following discharge.

Any charge tag processed during that two-day period will be included in the patient's bill.

Charges after the two-day audit period are _late_ and cannot be processed through the normal procedures. They must be presented to the business office, where a late (second) billing will be made. Late bills must show a minimum amount of $20.

Affected Departments

Reviewed _____

Subject	Effective Date	Latest Revision & Date
CLOSE-OUT FOR CHARGES	1-90	

At the end of each month or the fiscal year (June 30), all charges must be reconciled and processed to reflect accurately the revenue for that period.

All charge tags must be entered no later than 3P.M. on the last day of the period.

Affected Departments

Reviewed _____

Subject	Effective Date 1-90	Latest Revision & Date
INTERDEPARTMENTAL COST TRANSFERS		

Supplies transferred from one department to another department are charged to the department receiving and using the items. These item cost transfers are not for inventory items; they are for items already charged to a department being transferred to another department.

The cost transfers are allocated to the appropriate department's budget.

The interdepartmental cost transfer form (see sample) is used to record the transfer. The completed form is forwarded to accounting.

The interdepartmental cost transfer form can also be used as the supply order form and is prepared by the user department.

Affected Departments

Reviewed _____

INTERDEPARTMENTAL COST TRANSFER

DATE _____

| TRANSFER FROM: DEPARTMENT _____ | | COST CENTER # _____ | | | | |
| TRANSFER TO: DEPARTMENT _____ | | COST CENTER # _____ | | | | |

QUANTITY		CODE	DESCRIPTION	UNIT	UNIT/ COST	TOTAL
REQ'D	TRANS					
TOTAL QUANTITY DELIVERED					TOTAL COST	
REQUESTED BY			APPROVED BY			

ORIGINAL–TRANSFER FROM DEPARTMENT
Copy 1–Data Processing

SECTION XI

LINEN SERVICE
SECTION XI

Subject	Effective Date 1-90	Latest Revision & Date
LINEN SERVICE OVERVIEW		

Linen service is a function of materials management.

Its objective is to provide adequate amounts of clean linen to user departments on a scheduled basis and as needed.

Linen service is staffed from 6A.M. to 3:30P.M., 7 days a week. Backup is provided by dispatch after routine hours.

Service includes:

1. Coordinating linen processing with the contact laundry facility
2. Ensuring quality of clean linen processed
3. Sorting and distributing all clean linen
4. Controlling linen inventory
5. Distributing linen
6. Preparing soiled linen for return to the contact laundry facility
7. Repairing linen
8. Setting up linen packs

Affected Departments

Reviewed _____

Subject		Effective Date 1-90	Latest Revision & Date
CONTRACT LAUNDRY SERVICE			

Institutional linen is processed at a contract laundry facility.

The contract laundry processes linen under conditions acceptable by the State Health Department and the Joint Commission on Accreditation of Health Care Organizations.

The laundry charges the institution for linen processed on a <u>per-pound</u> basis. Linen is weighed soiled at the institution and clean at the laundry (<u>and</u> at the institution for a double-check). The price is based on an annually reviewed contract.

The laundry delivers clean linen and picks up soiled linen Monday through Saturday. It keeps clean linen separate from soiled and handles clean first.

Meetings are held monthly at the institution to discuss laundry service and any problems with the linen. Problems are noted so that there is a written record for the meeting. Action to be taken is followed up by the linen service supervisor.

The laundry processes linen according to the following formulas, which meet or exceed regulatory requirements:

Suds—break*	12 minutes	160 degrees	6-inch level
Bleach and Inex	10 minutes	150 degrees	6-inch level
Rinse	4 minutes	140 degrees	12-inch level
Rinse	4 minutes	120 degrees	12-inch level
Rinse	4 minutes	95 degrees	12-inch level
Sour-softener-bacteriastat	5 minutes	90 degrees	6-inch level

*OR and OB blue or green linen, same as above except 1 to 3 100-degree flushes, 4 minutes each at 12-inch level.

Affected Departments

Reviewed _____

Subject	Effective Date	Latest Revision & Date
SOILED LINEN HANDLING/CONTROL	1-90	

All soiled linen is bagged/contained so that employees can handle and transport it without risking contamination.

1. Soiled bed linen is removed from the bed and placed in the pillowcase. Any linen that will not fit in the pillowcase is placed in a plastic bag available from the Nurserver.

   Nonbed linen is added to the soiled pillowcase or plastic bag as needed.

   The bagged linen is placed immediately in the soiled (lower) section of the Nurserver or the closest linen hamper.

   Three times a day, housekeeping personnel remove the soiled linen from the Nurserver and transport it in a covered cart to the soiled utility room for transportation through the linen tube system to the soiled linen hold room at the dock. (Pickup times are 9A.M., 2:30P.M., and 8P.M.)

   If the soiled section of the Nurserver becomes full, nursing personnel contact housekeeping to make a special pickup. If they are unavailable, a supply technician is contacted. If he or she is unavailable, the nurse takes the soiled, bagged linen to the soiled utility room and places it in the utility cart or on the floor nearest the linen chute. Nursing personnel do not place bagged linen into the tube system. Only housekeeping and materials management personnel load the soiled linen into the system.

2. Ancillary departments (respiratory therapy, radiology, etc.) use linen bags in hamper frames. Linen must not be "overstuffed" into the bags, because they must fit into the 20-inch diameter tube system.

   Housekeeping personnel pick up the bagged, soiled linen and transport it to the soiled utility room for placement into the tube system. This is done on a scheduled basis.

   Departments requiring extra pickups should contact housekeeping.

   Pillowcases of soiled linen or linen bags should be placed in the tube system closed end first.

3. Isolation linen is placed in a water-soluble plastic bag, marked ISOLATION, and then placed into a red fabric bag. Isolation linen is processed in a separate load/formula at the laundry.

4. Precaution linen is handled the same as isolation linen.

5. Radioactive linen is bagged and retained in nuclear medicine/radiology until it is determined by the radiology supervisor to be safe to handle.

6. Surgery linen is bagged in a green fabric bag and taken to the linen hold room in a plastic-lined cart by housekeeping personnel. When surgery linen reaches the laundry, it is processed in a separate load/formula.

Affected Departments

Reviewed _____

Subject	Effective Date	Latest Revision & Date
SOILED LINEN HANDLING/CONTROL (cont.)	1-90	

7. <u>Bagged, soiled linen</u> is placed into the tube system and automatically transported to the <u>soiled linen hold room</u> at the receiving dock. There, the bags are placed into plastic-lined carts, and the plastic is placed over the top of the bagged linen to protect the environment from any bacteria. The carts remain in the hold room until picked up by the laundry. <u>Housekeeping</u> notifies <u>dispatch</u> by telephone or intercom when placing linen in the tube system. Dispatch notifies <u>receiving</u> so the carts may be moved into position in the hold room and a pileup of soiled linen is avoided.

<u>Monday through Saturday</u>, the laundry picks up the hampers of soiled linen at the dock. Hampers are weighed and the weight recorded so that records can be kept of how much soiled linen is sent out to compare with clean linen that is returned. Soiled linen weighs about 8 to 12 percent more than clean. The laundry returns linen in three working days. The weight of the soiled linen sent out can then be compared with the clean linen delivered.

8. <u>When handling soiled linen</u> at the <u>dock</u>, the following must be observed:

   a. The doors to receiving, the kitchen, and processed stores must be kept closed.
   b. The air curtain/blower must be left <u>off</u> while stacking soiled linen in the carts to prevent blowing of bacteria. The blower should be turned <u>on</u> when the garage door is opened while loading the linen onto the truck. The door to the hold room should be <u>closed</u> during this operation.
   c. <u>All personnel</u> handling the soiled linen that has come out of the bags or pillowcases must wear:

      (1) Jumpsuit or scrub gown (which is closed or tied together after use)
      (2) Disposable gloves
      (3) Shoe covers
      (4) Mask
      (5) Protective goggles

NOTE: All single-use/disposable items must be disposed of after each use.

Affected Departments

Reviewed _____

Subject	Effective Date	Latest Revision & Date
RECEIVING CLEAN LINEN	1-90	

Clean linen is received Monday through Saturday between 7 and 7:30 A.M. from the laundry.

Linen is delivered in plastic-lined clean hampers, covered, sorted, and pressed. Clean is always separate from soiled linen.

On receipt, linen hampers are counted, weighed, and recorded on the weekly linen report. These reports are kept, totaled at the end of the month, and compared with the laundry invoice received. (See sample.)

Linen is transported to the linen room, where it is removed from the hampers, sorted, and put on shelves waiting for delivery to user departments. Where possible, clean linen is loaded directly onto carts destined for user departments to avoid double handling.

At that time, inspection is made and the weekly linen report is completed, recording any problems or shortages. (See sample.)

This report is reviewed at the monthly meeting with the contract laundry facility.

Affected Departments

Reviewed _____

Page 1 of 1

INSTITUTIONAL LAUNDRY

INVOICE #20661

NAME	
ADDRESS	

SPECIAL INSTRUCTIONS	
ROUTE	
DAY	

↑

Pay only
last amount
in this column

WEEKLY LINEN REPORT

For the Week Ending _____

	Monday / Date	Tuesday / Date	Wednesday / Date	Thursday / Date	Friday / Date	Saturday / Date	Total / Date
Linen received:							
Housekeeping # carts/ total pounds							
Dietary # carts/ total pounds							
General linen # carts/ total pounds							
Grand total (clean) received # carts/ total pounds							
Linen sent:							
Housekeeping # carts/ total pounds							
Dietary # carts/ total pounds							
General linen # carts/ total pounds							
Rewash — total pounds (no charge)							
Stained — total pounds (extra charge)							
Grand total (soiled) sent # carts/ total pounds							
Processed by							

Subject	Effective Date 1-90	Latest Revision & Date
SORTING CLEAN LINEN		

All linen is received cleaned and sorted.

If the linen is not sorted, linen handlers sort it by type, put it away, and note the lack of sorting on the weekly linen report.

Continuous sorting problems are reviewed with the laundry at the monthly meeting or as frequently as needed.

Affected Departments

Reviewed _____

Subject LINEN INSPECTION/REPAIRS	Effective Date 1-90	Latest Revision & Date

All clean linen received is inspected to see that it is clean, pressed, sorted, and free from tears, holes, etc.

Items that are not clean or pressed properly are returned to the laundry for reprocessing.

Torn items are repaired by the institution's mender. Patched linen is inspected on the light table for additional holes or weak spots.

Repairs are made with a heat/pressure spot patcher. Enough overlap must be provided so that the holes will not "run" past the patch.

Linen that is repaired or patched too often is not an effective barrier for bacteria and must not be used.

Linen that is beyond repair or has more than four repair patches is taken out of circulation and used for rags or other purposes.

Affected Departments

Reviewed _____

Page 1 of 1

Subject	Effective Date 1-90	Latest Revision & Date
LINEN PACKS		

Packs of linen are assembled in the linen pack room and are further processed in the material processing area. Packs are sterilized according to accepted sterilization procedures.

Packs are made up according to a predetermined Kardex file that is updated at least annually or as changes occur. Changes are authorized by the user department and the area supervisor.

All linen is inspected, delinted, and repaired in this area also.

Affected Departments

Reviewed _____

Subject	Effective Date 1-90	Latest Revision & Date
INFECTION CONTROL FOR LINEN SERVICE		

In all instances, there is a strict separation of clean and soiled linen.

The laundry takes periodic microbiology cultures to an independent laboratory. Results are reported to the hospital.

In addition, the hospital's infection control officer conducts periodic inspections of the laundry plant and processes independent microbiology cultures on a random basis.

Scrub clothing is worn by all linen technicians and is changed daily. Proper hand-washing technique is followed by all linen personnel.

Soiled linen is contained during transport in carts or in the tube system.

Affected Departments

Reviewed _____

Subject LINEN INVENTORY CONTROL	Effective Date 1-90	Latest Revision & Date

Linen is delivered to all user departments on a quota basis—the required quantity for the next 24-hour period. This quantity is delivered automatically every 24 hours on either an exchange cart or in bulk.

Periodic inventory is taken of all linen in circulation (at the institution <u>and</u> at the laundry).

Inventories are taken on Mondays, so that all linen in circulation is accounted for. The laundry assists with this count.

The results of the inventories are compared with expected daily use to obtain the proper mix/balance of all linen items. Since the standard level is established at "7 par," there should be a proportionate number of each item in circulation. For example, if 500 washcloths are used daily (per the usage data), then there should be a total of 3,500 washcloths in circulation. If there is a lesser amount, more inventory is added. If there is an excess, washcloths are removed from circulation so that the balance is maintained.

The "7 par" standard is determined by noting the number of places throughout the system where linen may be:

Par 1—in use
Par 2—in patient's room
Par 3—in stock in user department
Par 4—in stock in linen service
Par 5—soiled at the institution
Par 6—soiled at the laundry
Par 7—in transit

In addition, linen delivered to user departments and linen returned is recorded (by weight and periodically by item count) and compared with that processed by the laundry.

Linen quotas for user departments are reviewed and adjusted as needed or at least semiannually to make sure they meet institutional requirements.

Affected Departments

Reviewed _____

Subject	Effective Date	Latest Revision & Date
CLEAN LINEN DISTRIBUTION	1-90	

The following linen delivery schedule is carried out daily (or as designated):

<u>Daily</u>—all carts are exchanged between 3 and 4P.M.

    Nursing units:
        Pediatrics
        4 north
        4 south
        3 north
        3 south
        2 north
        2 south
        CCU
        SICU

<u>Monday—Friday only:</u> 9 to 10:30A.M.

    All other user departments and bulk linen orders

<u>Special deliveries:</u>

    Extra linen required should be noted on the stock requisition and forwarded to linen service. These orders will be handled on a first come, first served basis and will be coordinated with scheduled deliveries (which have first priority).

<u>Emergency linen:</u>

    Can be obtained by telephoning dispatch

Affected Departments

Reviewed _____

Page 1 of 1

Subject	Effective Date 1-90	Latest Revision & Date
NEW LINEN		

All new linen put into circulation must be marked as institutional property.

A label is attached to each piece of linen with a heat-sensitive stamp. It includes the institution's name and address.

Items that have been in circulation long enough that the stamp has become faded should be restamped to avoid loss.

New linen should not be put into circulation without the approval of the supervisor or director.

Affected Departments

Reviewed _____

Page 1 of 1

Subject	Effective Date 1-90	Latest Revision & Date
PROCESSING CAFETERIA LINEN		

The commercial dry cleaner will process fine cafeteria linen (tablecloths, etc.). A contract is set up to handle this arrangement.

The dry cleaner picks up, processes, and returns the linen in about three (3) working days.

When dietary has linen ready for washing:

1. It is bagged in a clear plastic bag.
2. A list is made of what is to be processed (to avoid losses) and recorded on a nonstock request for purchasing services form.
3. The list is marked with the expected/required return date.
4. Linen service is called for pickup.

Linen service will:

1. Pick up bagged linen and request form
2. Mark outside the bag—DIETARY LINEN
3. Take it to the soiled receiving dock door
4. Call the dry cleaner to arrange for pickup

On return, the clean linen is delivered to dietary by linen service personnel.

If linen is not acceptably processed, linen service should contact the dry cleaner.

Affected Departments

Reviewed _____

Subject		Effective Date 1-90	Latest Revision & Date
	CHAPEL LINEN		

Chapel linen is processed by the commercial dry cleaner.

Linen personnel must contact the dry cleaner to arrange pickup of the items.

The nonstock request for purchasing services form should list all items and quantities to be processed and any special instructions.

When the linen has been returned, linen service picks it up and returns it to the chapel.

Affected Departments

Reviewed _____

Page 1 of 1

Subject		Effective Date	Latest Revision & Date
SPECIAL LINEN REQUESTS		1-90	

Departments requiring special linen processing or the makeup of special items by the linen mender must request such services in writing.

All details and specifications must be provided, or the request will be returned without action.

When the request has been completed, linen service will arrange for delivery or pickup of the item(s).

Affected Departments

Reviewed _____

Subject		Effective Date 1-90	Latest Revision & Date
STAINED LINEN			

Stained linen is linen that has been processed but contains a noticeable and unsightly discoloration or distinguishing mark.

When linen is received from the laundry, all stained linen is placed in a bag located in a cart/hamper set aside for stained linen. The bag is to be marked STAINED.

Stained linen, which is handled in a specific way by the laundry, should not be confused with "rewash" linen.

When a full cart/hamper has been accumulated, it should be returned to the laundry for processing, identified as STAINED.

The hospital pays for reprocessing of stained linen.

If repeated reprocessing of stained linen is unsuccessful, the linen is removed from circulation and used for rags.

Affected Departments

Reviewed _____

Subject		Effective Date 1-90	Latest Revision & Date
	REWASH LINEN		

When clean linen is received from the laundry, it is sorted and stored on racks until used to set up orders and carts.

"Rewash" is linen not properly processed; it is still soiled but not <u>stained</u> (e.g., feces on a sheet, sputum or any other foreign material on an item).

When a "rewash" item is discovered:

1. It is put aside in a linen bag located in a cart/hamper designated for REWASH.
2. At the end of the day, all rewash linen is weighed, and the weight is deducted from the clean linen delivered by the laundry on the next delivery day.
3. The rewash is noted on the institution's copy of the weekly linen report form.
4. The full bag of rewash linen is returned to the laundry for processing on the next day's pickup.

The hospital is not charged for rewash.

Affected Departments

Reviewed _____

Subject	Effective Date	Latest Revision & Date
CHARGES FOR LINEN USE	1-90	

To maintain accountability for linen usage and costs, user departments are "charged" for linen used on a per piece/pound basis. This includes the cost per pound charged by the laundry. It does not include any handling charge or the cost of the linen purchased.

On a daily basis, the number of linen items dispensed to each user area is recorded. The weight of each item is known. At the end of each period, the total quantity issued is multiplied by the weight per item. This total is multiplied by the cost per pound and charged to the user departments.

The total weight/charge per department is forwarded to accounting for allocation to the general ledger and appropriate budget account monthly.

Affected Departments

Reviewed _____

SECTION XII

PRINT SHOP
SECTION XII

Subject	Effective Date	Latest Revision & Date
PRINT SHOP OVERVIEW	1-90	

The print shop is open from 7:30A.M. to 4:30P.M., Monday through Friday, for large-volume special printing and duplicating services.

Personnel are to use the copying/duplicating equipment for official business only. These machines are not used for personal business, even on a fee basis.

Special types of copying/duplicating are produced on the print shop duplicator or press. A request for copying/duplicating form is to be filled out by the requesting party and sent to the print shop for service. (See sample.)

Problems with any of the auxiliary copy machines should be brought to the attention of the key operator (Monday through Friday, days—the print shop clerk; weekends and evenings—the copy machine service technician). Phone numbers for the key operators are posted on each machine.

Only trained, authorized personnel should attempt to solve problems with the equipment.

Copies that are ruined because of equipment malfunction should be placed in the "scrap" boxes provided. The institution obtains credit for any such copies.

Affected Departments

Reviewed _____

Subject		Effective Date 1-90	Latest Revision & Date
COPY MACHINES			

Copy machines are to be used for official business by in-house personnel only.

Copy machines are operated <u>only</u> with an <u>autotron key.</u> This is a coded device that, when inserted, activates the copy machine to operate and also automatically registers the number of copies on the counter contained in the autotron key. This number is used as a billing mechanism for departments.

User departments are "charged" for the number of copies they make according to the recording on the autotron key. The cost per copy does not include labor or overhead.

Auxiliary machines are used for making 1 to 20 copies of a single document. The copies are to be made by the department's own personnel. The print shop clerk does not provide this service.

More than 20 copies of any one document, sets, books, etc., should be made by the print shop clerk on the duplicating equipment in the print shop.

Problems with any of the copiers should be brought to the attention of the print shop clerk or the key operator on duty.

Affected Departments

Reviewed _____

Subject	Effective Date	Latest Revision & Date
DUPLICATING SERVICE	1-90	

The print shop provides duplicating service (printing and mimeographing) for a volume of 20 or more of any single original.

This includes hole punching, collating, etc.

Work to be duplicated is handled on a first come, first served basis and should be presented to the print shop clerk in "ready-to-print" condition. Adequate lead time must be allowed.

A request for copying/duplicating form (see sample) is filled out whenever this service is requested.

When the duplicating service is completed, the print shop notifies the requesting department to arrange for delivery or pickup.

User departments are charged for this service based on cost per copy. The print shop lists the quantity and cost per department on a report submitted to accounting each month for allocation to the general ledger and departmental budget accounts.

Affected Departments

Reviewed _____

Page 1 of 1

REQUEST FOR COPYING/DUPLICATING

DATE REQUESTED _____ DEPARTMENT _____

DATE REQUIRED _____ REQUESTED BY _____

===

NUMBER OF COPIES _____ SIZE   5½ x 8½ _____   3 x 5 _____

NUMBER OF SETS _____   8½ x 11 _____   4 x 6 _____

PAPER COLOR   White ____   Green ____   OTHER _____
              Blue ____   Pink ____
              Yellow ____ Cherry ____ PUNCHED 3-hole ____ STAPLED ____
              Salmon ____ Lilac ____   2-hole ____
              Goldenrod ____ Grey ____   Top ____
              Avocado ____ Beige ____   Side ____

PADDED ____   UNPADDED ____   PAD SIZE 50 ____   100 ____   COLLATED ____

SPECIAL INSTRUCTIONS _____

_____

===

DATE COMPLETED _____ COMPLETED BY _____

DATE PICKED UP _____ RECEIVED BY _____

Subject	Effective Date	Latest Revision & Date
STOCK (INVENTORY) FORMS	1-90	

The print shop prints a variety of forms used throughout the institution and stored in the storeroom as inventory. Each item is handled like any stock item. It has a unique stock number, reorder point and quantity, unit of measure, etc.

Purchasing considers the print shop to be a "vendor," therefore it submits a purchase order listing which forms to print and how many of each.

Once forms are completed, the print shop indicates the quantity printed on the purchase order and forwards the finished forms to the storeroom where they are received. The purchase order is returned to purchasing to signify that the order is completed and received. The records must be updated to reflect this.

The print shop maintains a numerical file (by form number) of all masters (originals) of forms printed in the print shop.

Obsolete forms are cut and padded for scratch paper by the print shop and distributed to user departments at no cost.

Affected Departments

Reviewed _____

Page 1 of 1

Subject	Effective Date 1-90	Latest Revision & Date
NONSTOCK FORMS		

Nonstock (noninventory) forms are run in the print shop as a duplicating service.

The request for copying/duplicating form should be filled out by each department and presented to the print shop with the master (original).

Adequate lead time (at least three business days) is necessary, as the print shop handles a variety of orders.

Copies of the masters are filed in the print shop by department number. Forms are numbered for identification. The number consists of the department (cost center) number, followed by the number of that form in that department (e.g., 600-1, 600-2, 600-3, and so on for forms in nursing service, department #600). The original or revision date is placed in the lower left corner of the form.

Affected Departments

Reviewed _____

Page 1 of 1

Subject	Effective Date	Latest Revision & Date
EQUIPMENT MAINTENANCE	1-90	

The print shop maintains current operating manuals on all copy, duplicating, and other related equipment.

The print shop equipment is maintained on a routine basis by the print shop clerk. This includes cleaning, filling supplies, clearing jams, etc.

Major or preventive maintenance is performed by an authorized technician from outside vendors. This is either prescheduled according to a contract with the company or on an emergency basis when called for by the print shop clerk.

Records of all maintenance are kept for each piece of equipment to provide information on equipment or service reliability.

Affected Departments

Reviewed _____

Page 1 of 1

Subject		Effective Date	Latest Revision & Date
EQUIPMENT OPERATION		1-90	

Jogger:

The jogger straightens stacks of paper by jogging them into order. This machine requires no maintenance, but it must <u>only</u> be operated when there is paper in it.

Electric stapler:

The electric stapler is operated by plugging it in, turning the switch to the "on" position, and inserting the material into the stapler. When the paper hits the "staple guides," a staple is released. To load the stapler, turn switch to "off," press button to load, insert staples, and close lid. Return switch to "on" and resume stapling.

Laminator:

To operate the laminator, remove the cover, insert the plug, and put the plate in operating position. There are three lights on this machine: "on/off," "preheat," and "ready." To use the laminator, push the button to "preheat" until the "ready" light comes on. Then push the button to "on"; the rollers will start revolving. Place the material to be laminated on the plate until the rollers start to grab it. When it is completely out the other end, make sure to leave at least two inches of plastic out of the machine so that the material won't roll back into the machine. To continue laminating, push the button back to "preheat" to keep the machine hot, but stop the rollers. When finished, press the "off" button. This shuts off both the machine <u>and</u> the rollers. Replace the plate, unplug the cord, and put the cover back on.

Folding machine:

To operate the folding machine, remove the cover and insert the plug. On the machine, there is a "chart for standard folds" that tells where to place the guides. There are two guides, one at the top and one on the side of the machine. Take the removable plate and hook onto the bar at the end of the machine. When these are set, fan the paper to be folded so that the top paper is the first one to enter the machine. Turn the machine "on." The rollers in front will grab the paper and fold it in the style selected. The only care this machine requires is replacing the removable plate, unplugging the cord, and replacing the cover.

Table-top offset duplicator:

For operating instructions, see the manufacturer's manual.

Affected Departments

Reviewed _____

Subject	Effective Date	Latest Revision & Date
SCRAP COPIES	1-90	

Copies destroyed because of equipment malfunctions are reimbursed by the company that owns/leases or services the machines for the healthcare institution.

A "scrap" box is located near each machine. When copies are ruined, they should be placed in the box. The box is collected by the company service technician each month, and the institution receives appropriate credit.

Affected Departments

Reviewed _____

Subject	Effective Date 1-90	Latest Revision & Date
INVOICE APPROVAL		

The hospital receives an invoice each month for equipment that it leases or rents for copying or duplicating.

The copy volumes shown on the invoice must be verified by comparing them with the logs. The meter readings also are compared with the invoice and the log.

The invoice and subsequent logs are reviewed by the purchasing manager and, on review and reconciliation, are authorized for payment by the purchasing manager's signature.

The invoice is forwarded to accounting for payment.

Problems or discrepancies are fully investigated by the purchasing manager before payment is made.

Affected Departments

Reviewed _____

Subject	Effective Date 1-90	Latest Revision & Date
PRINT SHOP SUPPLIES		

The print shop clerk is responsible for maintaining all supplies necessary for operations in the department. This includes paper, ink, toner, etc.

Supplies obtained from the storeroom are ordered as scheduled (weekly) on a stock requisition. The print shop clerk is authorized to order these items.

Nonstock or direct supplies from outside vendors must be ordered on a nonstock request for purchasing services form and forwarded to the purchasing manager for approval.

Any equipment needs or requests must be authorized by the director of materials management.

Affected Departments

Reviewed _____

SECTION XIII

MAIL ROOM
SECTION XIII

Subject	Effective Date 1-90	Latest Revision & Date
MAIL ROOM OVERVIEW		

The mail room is responsible for all outgoing mail and all incoming U.S. mail processing.

The mail room is open Monday through Friday from 8A.M. to 4:30P.M. for outgoing and incoming mail.

Interhospital mail is placed in the pneumatic tube system (PTS) from sending to receiving departments. Other items are delivered by each department or placed in the destination department's mail box in the mail room.

Incoming mail is picked up from the post office at 8:30A.M. daily by materials management.

Incoming mail is distributed via the PTS. Packages too large to fit in the PTS are delivered by distribution personnel with supply orders. Departments are notified by telephone/intercom when packages arrive.

Outgoing mail must be prepared properly before it is presented to the mail room for processing.

All mail room equipment is to be operated by mail room staff only.

Personal mail is not handled by the mail room. All personal mail should be deposited in the mail box at the main entrance to the facility.

Affected Departments

Reviewed _____

Page 1 of 1

Subject		Effective Date 1-90	Latest Revision & Date
	INCOMING MAIL		

Mail is picked up by a designated person in materials management at the U.S. Post Office at 8:30A.M., Monday through Friday.

The mail is sorted and distributed by mail room personnel.

All incoming mail is sorted into two categories:

1. Patient mail is sorted in alphabetical order. The auxiliary/volunteers pick up patient mail in the mail room each day at 11A.M. and deliver it to the patients in their rooms.

2. Business mail is sorted in department mail boxes. Small letters and items are sent directly to the departments via the PTS. Departments without a PTS station have their mail sent to the closest station (as agreed on by the department).

   Mail and packages that are too large to fit in the PTS (6 inches × 15 inches) are delivered by distribution personnel once each day, with stock or other supply orders.

This service is not provided on weekends or holidays.

Affected Departments

Reviewed _____

Subject	Effective Date 1-90	Latest Revision & Date
OUTGOING MAIL		

All outgoing letters, packages, etc., must be in the mail room by 10:45A.M. Mail should be sent there via the PTS or, if too large, delivered.

All mail must have the following <u>typed</u> information:

1. Name
2. Address
3. City and state
4. Zip code
5. Return address

All hospital mail must be stamped. The mail room will use the automatic postage machine to affix appropriate postage.

Affected Departments

Reviewed _____

Subject	Effective Date	Latest Revision & Date
INTERDEPARTMENTAL MAIL DISTRIBUTION	1-90	

Mail is distributed between institutional departments via the PTS and by a mail room box system.

Departments that do not have their own PTS stations arrange for the mail room and all other departments to send mail to the closest PTS station.

It is each department's responsibility to see that its interdepartmental mail is delivered to or received from other departments. If a PTS is unavailable or incapable of handling such items, they must be delivered by the departments involved.

Mail not distributed through the PTS is taken to the mail room by the sending department. Mail is placed in the destination departments' mail boxes or slots by the sender. Departments are expected to check mail boxes periodically to collect mail.

Affected Departments

Reviewed _____

Subject	Effective Date	Latest Revision & Date
MAIL ROOM EQUIPMENT OPERATION	1-90	

Refer to equipment brochures for correct operation of all equipment.

Affected Departments

Reviewed _____

SECTION XIV

MATERIAL PROCESSING
SECTION XIV

Subject	Effective Date	Latest Revision & Date
MATERIAL PROCESSING OVERVIEW	1-90	

Materials management is responsible for reprocessing all reusables used throughout the institution for patient care. These reusables include: surgical instruments, basins, and other patient utensils; carts; dishware; sterile linen; and movable patient care equipment, including respiratory therapy type.

Hours of operation are 7A.M. to 11P.M. daily.

All items processed follow a strict traffic pattern of soiled to clean. The soiled areas are physically separated from the clean, and all items entering the soiled area are processed before being moved to the clean area. They are "decontaminated" and rendered safe for handling/use or for further processing (terminal sterilization).

Equipment used for processing is the "pass-through" type to facilitate the soiled-to-clean flow.

All environmental conditions in the processing department are monitored for quality and acceptability (temperature, residual ethylene oxide [ETO], humidity, air pressure and changes, etc.). Equipment is also monitored mechanically, chemically, and biologically and is subject to ongoing preventive maintenance. All regulatory guidelines are met or exceeded.

Personnel are formally trained for operating the equipment and performing departmental tasks. Performance is evaluated on a regular basis. Dress code and traffic patterns are controlled to prevent cross-contamination.

A limited number of items are not processed by materials management. These specialty items, processed by the department responsible for them, include: instruments owned by private surgeons, air-powered instruments, extremely delicate eye and ear instruments, and limited specialty items so designated.

All items handled by materials management are processed with the newest, most efficient and effective techniques and equipment available.

A surgical case cart system is used to transport the supplies, linens, and instruments to surgery and to return them for reprocessing.

Affected Departments

Reviewed _____

Subject		Effective Date 1-90	Latest Revision & Date
QUALITY CONTROL OF IN-HOUSE STERILIZATION			

1. Identification of the wrappers and shelf life of sterile items processed in the institution

   A sterile item must be packaged in the appropriate wrapper to maintain sterility through its intended shelf life.

   a. Each kind of packaging and processing method has a specific shelf life (i.e., the length of time an item is considered sterile if unopened).

   (1) Items with a shelf life of 30 days are to be double-wrapped in water-resistant, nonwoven wrappers* and color-coded to indicate the method of sterilization to be used:

      (a) Buff color for steam

      (b) Green color for gas

      *Muslin wrappers may be used in double thickness if nonwoven wrappers are unavailable.

   (2) Items with a shelf life of 180 days are to be double-wrapped in nonwoven wrappers, taped with the appropriate color tape, and sterilized. Following steam sterilization and cooling to room temperature, these items are to be placed in a plastic bag (minimum thickness 3mil) and heat sealed.

   (3) Items with a shelf life of 365 days are to be placed in a peel pack (pouches or tubes, one side of surgical-grade paper and the other side of 1.5mm polypropylene and 0.5mil Mylar) and heat sealed on side edges.

   b. Each pack prepared for sterilization should be labeled with the load number, expiration date, name of item(s) in the pack, and initials of the person who prepared that pack.

   In use, this labeling tape contains all the important information and should be saved by the person who opens the pack until the pack is used. Any problems relevant to the pack can be communicated to the person or department responsible for its processing if the labeling tape is available for analysis.

Affected Departments

Reviewed _____

Subject	Effective Date	Latest Revision & Date
QUALITY CONTROL OF IN-HOUSE STERILIZATION (cont.)	1-90	

2. <u>Preparation of packs and trays to be terminally sterilized</u>

All packs are to be prepared with: a filled out steam or gas chemical indicator strip, then wrapped and taped with steam tape or gas tape. Each pack is to be dated with the seven-digit identifying <u>load number</u> (e.g., 2 01 14 03—2 is the sterilizer number; 01 is the month, January; 14 is the day of the month; 03 is the third load sterilized on 1/14). The expiration date appropriate to the type of wrapper is also indicated. This information is on a tag that is placed on the labeling tape closest to the name of the item. (See sample of load # tag.)

Sterilizer monitor record cards must be made out for each load sterilized and saved in a file in the department doing the sterilizing (materials management). (See sample.)

a. Steam sterilizer:

(1) Obtain one indicator strip for each pack or tray. Sterilizer tape may be used when a loose indicator strip is undesirable.

(2) Place this strip in every pack or tray prepared for sterilization.

(3) Prepare tape with tag including load number and expiration date, name of item(s), and operator's initials.

NOTE: Those departments that do their own wrapping do not put the load number on the tape. This is done before loading into the sterilizer by materials management.

(4) Wrap pack or tray and tape with steam sterilizer tape (buff color).

(5) Load sterilizer with all packs or trays to be sterilized.

(6) When sterilizer is loaded, a sterilizer monitor record card must be placed in the center of each load after the following information is filled in:

(a) Date—month, day, year
(b) Sterilizer number
(c) Load number
(d) Load contents—list departments and number of packs for each department
(e) Total number of items (bundles) in the load
(f) Operator's full signature—first and last name
(g) Expiration date

A piece of sterilizer tape is put on the card in its designated place.

NOTE: If there are different wrappers, see the back of the card to indicate expiration dates.

(7) Run sterilizer through complete cycle.

Affected Departments

Reviewed _____

LOAD # TAG

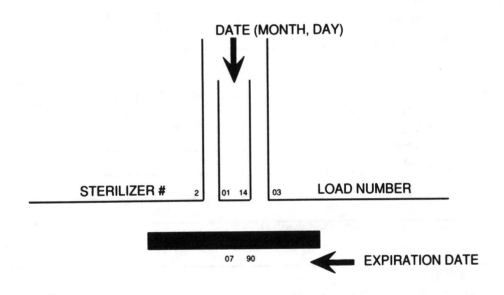

STERILIZER MONITOR RECORD CARD

CYCLE ☐ STEAM
        STERILIZER # _____

    ETO GAS ☐
    WARM CYCLE ☐
    COLD CYCLE ☐

PLACE
INDICATOR
TAPE
STRIP
HERE

      RECORDING CHART # _____

DATE
LOAD #

PLACE LOAD
LABEL HERE

EXPIRATION DATE _____

(MONTH)   (DAY)   (YEAR)

LOAD ITEM TOTAL
_____

DEPARTMENTS 1. _____   2. _____   3. _____

                 4. _____   5. _____   6. _____

_____   _____

(OPERATOR'S SIGNATURE)   (DEPARTMENT)

BOWIE-DICK TEST   CULTURE
    ☐ POSITIVE   ☐ NEGATIVE   ☐ POSITIVE   ☐ NEGATIVE

Subject	Effective Date 1-90	Latest Revision & Date
QUALITY CONTROL OF IN-HOUSE STERILIZATION (cont.)		

(8) When sterilizer cycle is complete, remove record card first. If the entire chemical indicator turned brown, it means conditions for sterilization have been met, and the sterilizer can be unloaded. (If the complete color change has not taken place, contact the manager so that measures can be taken to find the problem. DO NOT RELEASE THIS LOAD TO THE INSTITUTION FOR USE.)

(9) The sterilizer monitor record card is filed as a permanent reference and legal record. It is kept for seven (7) years.

(10) Unload sterilizer and release the packs for in-house use.

b. ETO gas sterilizer

(1) Obtain one gas chemical indicator strip for each pack or tray. Sterilizer tape may be used when a loose indicator strip is undesirable.

(2) Place this strip in every pack or tray prepared for sterilization.

(3) Prepare tape and tag, which includes load number and expiration date, identification of item(s), and operator's initials.

NOTE: Those departments that do their own wrapping do not put the load number on the tape. This is done before loading by materials management.

(4) Wrap each pack or tray and tape with gas tape (green color).

(5) Load gas sterilizer with all packs or trays to be sterilized.

(6) When sterilizer is loaded, a sterilizer monitor record card must be placed in the center of each load after completing the following information:

(a) Date—month, day, year
(b) Sterilizer number
(c) Load number
(d) Load contents—list departments and number of packs for each department
(e) Total number of items (bundles) in the load
(f) Operator's full signature—first and last name
(g) Expiration date

A piece of sterilizer tape is put on the card in the designated place.

NOTE: If there are different wrappers, see the back of the card to indicate expiration dates.

Affected Departments

Reviewed _____

Subject	Effective Date	Latest Revision & Date
QUALITY CONTROL OF IN-HOUSE STERILIZATION (cont.)	1-90	

(7) A biological spore culture must be placed in every load.

(8) Run sterilizer through complete cycle.

(9) When cycle is complete, remove record card first. If the lines on the indicator turned red, it means conditions for sterilization have been met and the sterilizer can be unloaded. (If the color change has not completely appeared, contact the manager so that measures can be taken to find the problem. DO NOT RELEASE THIS LOAD TO THE INSTITUTION FOR USE.)

(10) The sterilizer monitor record card is filed as a permanent reference and legal record. It is kept for seven (7) years, or the minimum period required by law.

(11) Label the culture with the load number and department name.

(12) Unload sterilizer and properly aerate all items.

(13) Quarantine contents until a 24-hour negative reading of the culture is reported from the laboratory.

(14) Release the packs to the institution for use on receipt of the microbiology culture report. (See sample.) If a positive report is returned, see <u>Recall</u> information.

3. <u>Sterile items processed</u>

All sterile packs are to be checked for sterility by the <u>user</u> before they are used. All sterile packs will have a strip inside the pack to indicate whether sterilization conditions have been achieved throughout the pack. All sterile packs will have color tape on the outside of the pack to indicate that the items have been processed in a sterilizer. All sterile packs will have a load number to indicate the sterilizer load in which the pack was sterilized. All sterile packs will have the initials of the person who prepared and processed the pack. (See sample of load # tag.)

   a. <u>In-use</u> checking of sterility of packs:

     (1) Before opening the pack, check the expiration date to determine if the pack can be used, and check the tape to determine if the item was processed in a sterilizer:

       (a) Steam—buff tape with dark brown diagonal lines
       (b) Gas—green tape with red diagonal lines

     (2) When opening the pack, save the wrapper until the pack is used up so that any problems with the pack can be communicated to the processor.

Affected Departments

Reviewed _____

Procedure #14.2

MICROBIOLOGY REQUISITION/CULTURE REPORT

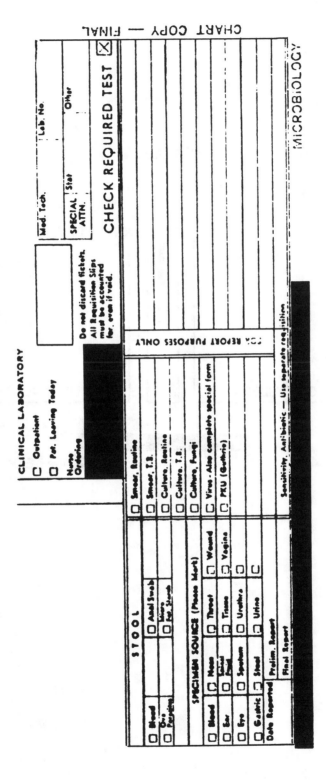

371

LOAD # TAG

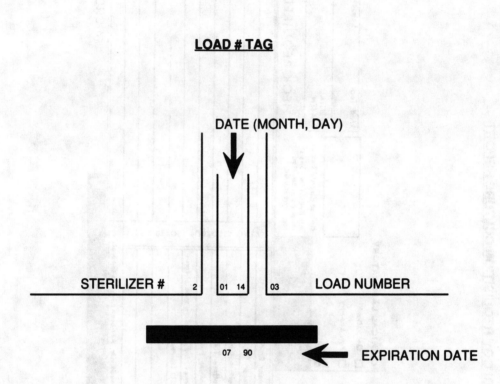

DATE (MONTH, DAY)

STERILIZER #   2   01 14   03   LOAD NUMBER

07   90   ◄—— EXPIRATION DATE

Subject	Effective Date	Latest Revision & Date
QUALITY CONTROL OF IN-HOUSE STERILIZATION (cont.)	1-90	

(3) After the pack is opened, check the strip inside to determine if conditions of sterilization were achieved throughout the pack:

    (a) Steam—dark brown stripe will be on the strip
    (b) Gas—dark red stripe will be on the strip

b. In-storage checking of sterility of packs:

(1) On Monday morning, an assigned person in each department that stores sterile supplies is to check all in-house-processed sterile packs to determine if shelf life has expired (date has been exceeded).

(2) The expiration date should not be earlier than the date of checking.

(3) The chemical indicator tape should show that the item was processed in a sterilizer:

    (a) Steam—buff tape with dark brown diagonal lines
    (b) Gas—green tape with red diagonal lines

(4) Items that have passed the expiration date should be returned to materials management for reprocessing.

4. Monitoring of sterilizers

All sterilizers are to be monitored chemically, biologically, and mechanically.

a. Chemical monitors: These are items that show by a chemical reaction (notably a color change) that they have been exposed to the conditions of sterilization.

(1) Strips (see sample of sterility indicator strip):

    (a) Steam—dark brown line
    (b) Gas—dark red line

(2) Tape (see sample of sterility indicator strip):

    (a) Steam—buff tape changes to dark brown diagonal stripes on a buff background
    (b) Gas—green tape changes to red diagonal lines on a green background

(3) Sterilizer monitor record cards (see sample):

    (a) Steam—dark brown line (indicator tape on each card)
    (b) Gas—red line (indicator tape on each card)

Affected Departments

Reviewed _____

Page 5 of 10

STERILIZER MONITOR RECORD CARD

CYCLE ☐ STEAM   ETO GAS   ☐   ┌─────────────┐
            STERILIZER # _____   WARM CYCLE ☐   │   PLACE   │
                                                  COLD CYCLE   ☐   │ INDICATOR │
      RECORDING CHART # _____   │   TAPE   │
DATE   │   STRIP   │
LOAD #   │   HERE   │
      ┌──────────────────────┐   └─────────────┘
      │   │   EXPIRATION DATE _____
      │   PLACE LOAD   │   (MONTH)   (DAY)   (YEAR)
      │   LABEL HERE   │   LOAD ITEM TOTAL
      │   │   _____
      └──────────────────────┘

DEPARTMENTS 1. _____   2. _____   3. _____

             4. _____   5. _____   6. _____

_____   _____
            (OPERATOR'S SIGNATURE)   (DEPARTMENT)

_____

BOWIE-DICK TEST   CULTURE
      ☐ POSITIVE   ☐ NEGATIVE   ☐ POSITIVE   ☐ NEGATIVE

Subject	Effective Date 1-90	Latest Revision & Date
QUALITY CONTROL OF IN-HOUSE STERILIZATION (cont.)		

(4) Bowie-Dick test sheet (see sample):

    (a) 9 inch × 11 inch sheets of paper impregnated with chemicals that change color when the conditions of sterilization have been met (shows absence of air pockets in vacuum sterilizer—steam only)

    (b) Vac/steam sterilizer only

(5) Sterilizer temperature recording chart (see sample): shows time and temperatures reached during cycle

b. Biological monitors: These are strips of paper that have been impregnated with bacterial spores. The bacterial spores will be killed if all the conditions of sterilization have been met.

    (1) Steam—brown cap ampules or spore strips/bacillus stearothermophillus
    (2) Gas—green cap ampules or spore strips/b-subtillus

c. Monitoring schedule:

    (1) Steam—sterilization of items effected by the use of steam under pressure. Parameters to be checked are vacuum, time, temperature, pressure, and concentration of steam.

        (a) Bowie-Dick test every day
        (b) Spore test every day (this includes flash sterilizers)

    (2) ETO gas—sterilization of items effected by the use of ethylene oxide, heat, and humidity. Parameters to be checked are vacuum, time, temperature, percent of humidity, and concentration of ethylene oxide gas.

        (a) Spore test every load

d. Monitoring procedure:

    (1) Chemical monitoring

        (a) Every morning, run each steam sterilizer through a complete cycle using the Bowie-Dick test.

        (b) Preparation and placement of the test pack:

           i) Bowie-Dick test sheet should be placed in the center of 36 standard towels to form a test pack or, as an alternate, in the largest and most dense (weight/volume) pack, which should have overall dimensions of approximately 12 inches × 12 inches × 20 inches and weigh no more than 12 pounds.

Affected Departments

Reviewed _____

BOWIE-DICK TEST SHEET

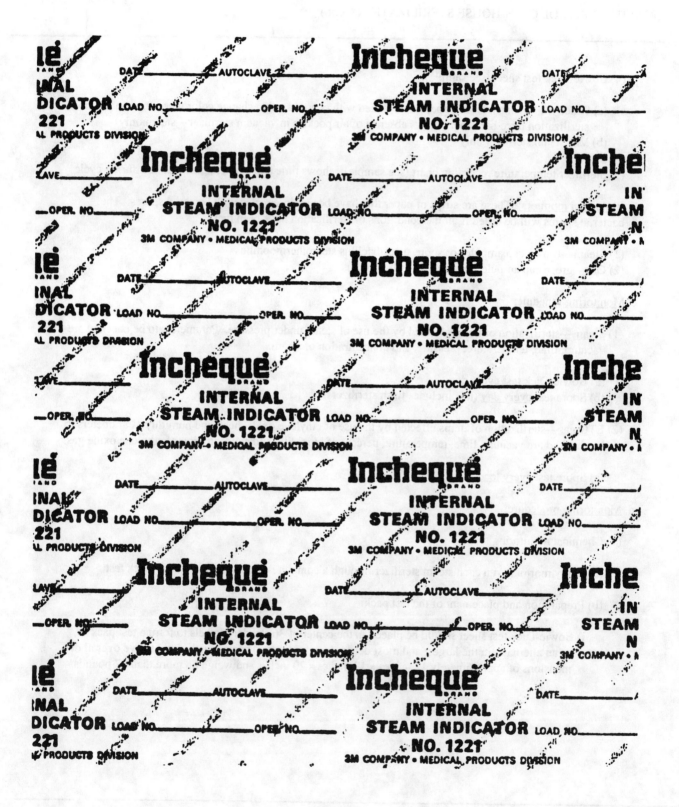

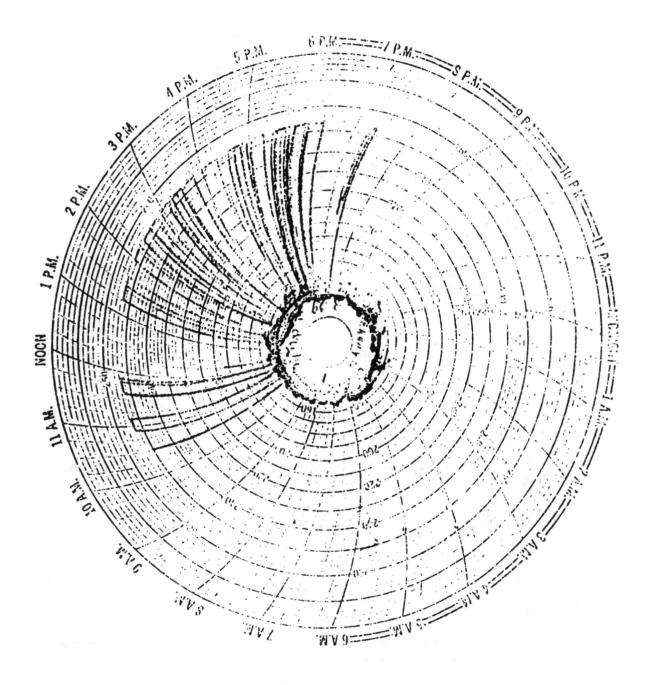

STERILIZER TEMPERATURE RECORDING CHART

Subject	Effective Date	Latest
QUALITY CONTROL OF IN-HOUSE STERILIZATION (cont.)	1-90	Revision & Date

ii) When testing a Hi-vac (high speed vacuum sterilizer), this test pack should be placed in the front bottom of an otherwise empty sterilizer. When testing a downward displacement (gravity) sterilizer, this test pack should be placed in the center of the sterilizer chamber. This must be the only pack in the sterilizer to ensure that any entrapped air does not exhibit itself in any pack other than the test pack.

iii) This test pack should be sterilized in the usual manner.

iv) The white center lines will turn dark brown after the cycle if all the air has been eliminated from the chamber of the sterilizer and the correct temperature has been achieved.

v) IMPORTANT: An incomplete or uneven color change indicates that the sterilizer is in need of repair.

vi) This system should be used every morning as the first sterilization cycle on each sterilizer, because the weakest point of daily sterilization is the first cycle. Daily use will determine if the sterilizer is operating properly.

(c) When the test pack has run the cycle, remove it, open the pack, and:

   i) Complete the bottom of the Bowie-Dick test sheet listing:

      a) Sterilizer number
      b) Load number
      c) Date—month, day, year
      d) Full-name signature in the operator section

   ii) If conditions for sterilization have been met (entire chemical indicator turns brown), file the report in a legal record file for that day's cycle

   iii) If a malfunction is detected, run the test again and report it immediately to the manager, who will initiate a recall on all items processed through the sterilizer the previous day, pending investigation

(d) This test is not used in the ETO gas sterilizer.

(2) Biological monitoring/steam sterilizing

(a) Every morning during the cycle that contains the Bowie-Dick test, a steam (brown cap) ampule or spore strip is to be placed in the sterilizer.

Affected Departments

Reviewed _____

Subject		Effective Date	Latest Revision & Date
QUALITY CONTROL OF IN-HOUSE STERILIZATION (cont.)		1-90	

(b) After the cycle is completed, remove the ampule, and label it with the load number, the date, and the department name. Match this test ampule with another ampule that has NOT been sterilized. This latter ampule is the control ampule for laboratory personnel. Label it with the date and department name.

(c) Deliver these two (2) ampules to the laboratory with a microbiology requisition/culture report (see sample) that has the department name, date, and load number for the test ampule and the department name and date for the control ampule. These ampules should be delivered to the laboratory at 8:30A.M. by the department that has "test run" the ampules.

(d) The laboratory will culture these ampules. Results of the cultures will be given after 24 hours of incubation. A final microbiology culture report will be given to the person delivering the new ampules the next day, so that recall of items processed can be initiated, if necessary.

(e) The laboratory and the departments that sterilize will keep records of all cultures.

(3) Biological monitoring/gas sterilizing

(a) Every load sterilized in the gas sterilizer must be monitored with a gas (green cap) ampule or spore strip.

(b) Label all test ampules with the load number and the department name. Send them immediately to the laboratory. Also send a control ampule (one that has NOT been sterilized) that has been labeled with the date and department name.

(c) The laboratory will culture these ampules. Results of the cultures will be given after 24 hours of incubation, and a final microbiology culture report will be given 48 hours after incubation. These reports will be given to the person delivering the new ampules the next day, so that recall of items processed can be initiated, if necessary.

(d) The laboratory and the departments that sterilize will keep records of all cultures.

(4) Biological culture system

(a) Remove indicators from sterilizer. Just before incubation, hold the capsule indicator upright and crush the glass ampule inside the plastic tube, with both thumbs and forefingers positioned half on the cap and half on the plastic tube.

(b) Check water temperature frequently. When properly operating, the water in incubator no. 107 (green) should be at 40°C; the water in incubator no. 106 (brown) should be at 56°C.

(c) Run unsterilized control test daily. Crush the glass ampule inside the plastic tube as described above in step a. After crushing, place the control indicator in the proper incubator. Check for growth after 24 hours. All control indicators should turn yellow.

Affected Departments

Reviewed _____

MICROBIOLOGY REQUISITION/CULTURE REPORT

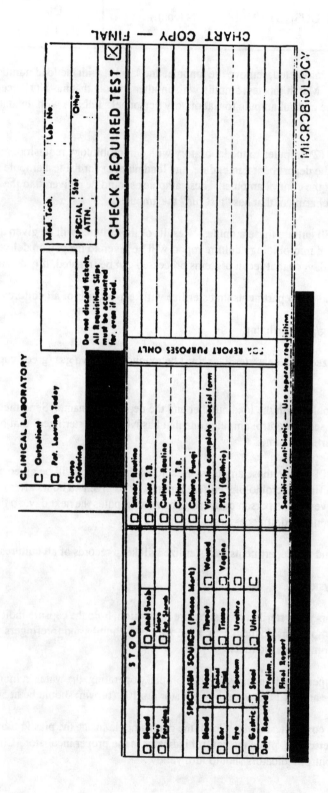

Subject	Effective Date	Latest Revision & Date
QUALITY CONTROL OF IN-HOUSE STERILIZATION (cont.)	1-90	

(d) After 24 and 48 hours, remove test indicators and check for growth. Longer incubation is not necessary nor recommended. Most positive cultures occur within 24 hours.

(e) Record results.

(f) If a positive result (yellow color) is observed, repeat test procedure using several indicators placed throughout the sterilizer. If results are again positive, contact maintenance to examine sterilizer to determine the cause of malfunction. It takes only one positive indicator to demonstrate marginal sterilizer performance.

(g) Avoid storing indicators near ETO or other volatile sterilizing agents.

(h) Dispose of positive indicators in the same manner as other microbiological waste.

5. Recall of items when a sterilizer has failed

When a Bowie-Dick test or a biological monitor show questionable sterility results, all items that were processed in the indicated sterilizer must be returned to processing so they can be reprocessed.

a. Upon receipt of a report that chemical (Bowie-Dick test) or biological indicators show that a sterilizer is malfunctioning, notify the manager immediately. If the Bowie-Dick test is positive, run it again. If it is still positive, notify the infection control officer and then:

b. IMMEDIATELY: Be sure "out of order" sign is placed on the sterilizer.

c. Call maintenance or the service department of the equipment manufacturer to arrange for repair of the sterilizer.

d. If packs or trays were in the load when indicators showed conditions for sterilization were not met, break these packs down to be prepared again, or contact the user departments to do this.

e. Check sterilizer monitor record cards to determine the last loads processed through the malfunctioning sterilizer.

f. Determine, from load numbers on sterilizer monitor record cards (see sample), which packs or trays were processed in loads where conditions for sterilization are questionable.

g. Immediately contact the departments involved with the load by telephone and advise them of the load number(s) in question. Then, all packs or trays clearly identified by the corresponding load number(s) are to be returned to processing to be reprocessed or are to be broken down and prepared again for sterilization.

h. Document the corrective steps taken on the sterilizer monitor record card in the sterilization records. This documentation must be detailed to allow anyone who looks at it to know exactly what happened, why it happened, and what was done to correct the problem. It must be signed with the operator's full sugnature and dated.

Affected Departments

Reviewed _____

STERILIZER MONITOR RECORD CARD

I. Expiration Date—Should be LATER or SAME as date of use

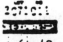
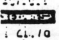

II. Outside Tape —Should show pack was in a sterilizer

Sterilized   *Not Sterilized*

A. Steam

B. Gas (Ethylene oxide)

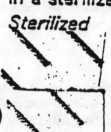

C.

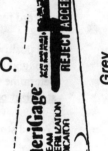

Sterilized

Grey

III. Inside Strip —Should show conditions for sterilization were met

Sterilized   *Not Sterilized*

A. Steam

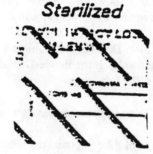
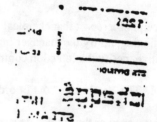

B. Gas (Ethylene oxide)

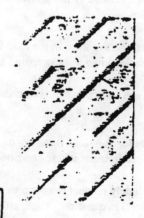

Sterilized

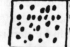

SteriGage Gas Sterilization Strip
When pattern appears, conditions for sterilization have been met

C.

Yellow

ONLY USE PACKS THAT FULFILL ALL THREE REQUIREMENTS

UNSTERILE PACKS MUST BE REPROCESSED
TO INSURE SAFETY FOR PATIENTS

Subject	Effective Date	Latest Revision & Date
QUALITY CONTROL OF IN-HOUSE STERILIZATION (cont.)	1-90	

6. <u>Records</u>

All records of the system are to be filed chronologically by day and kept together in the file for seven (7) years.

The records for each day's activities should include:

a. Bowie-Dick test sheet

b. Microbiology requisition/culture report(s)

c. Sterilizer monitor record card(s)

d. Sterilizer temperature recording chart

e. Any follow-up done on recalls

f. Records of cultures taken on disposable supplies or other items

7. <u>Monitoring of commercially sterilized/disposable supplies</u>

a. Because of liabilities that the hospital does not want to and should not assume, DISPOSABLE SUPPLIES WILL NOT BE STERILIZED FOR REUSE. They are disposed of after use or contamination with the rest of the institution's trash. This is also true for items that have reached the expiration date and have not been used (e.g., IV fluid).

b. If a manufacturer will state, in writing, that its product may be resterilized after use, the institution will <u>consider</u> resterilizing a disposable item. The manufacturer must state, in writing, that it assumes full liability for the product in case of a defect or breakdown in the quality of the item after reprocessing. The manufacturer must also state how many times, and by what method, reprocessing can be accomplished. Resterilization and reuse of disposables will be considered only if the product is unavailable in a timely or cost-effective manner in an <u>emergency.</u>

Affected Departments

Reviewed _____

Subject		Effective Date 1-90	Latest Revision & Date
OPERATING THE WASHER/STERILIZER			

The equipment used to process all hard goods (non-heat- or water-sensitive items) renders them completely safe for use or further processing.

When items have been accumulated for processing, select the proper basket and place all like items in that basket. Never load baskets too full because they will not fit into the machine or may hit moving parts in the chamber.

Operating instructions:

See equipment operating instruction manual.

If machine fails to operate, contact the manager or the maintenance department.

Affected Departments

Reviewed _____

Subject	Effective Date	Latest Revision & Date
OPERATING THE CART WASHER	1-90	

All carts used to transport soiled items to the decontamination area are cleaned in the cart washer before being used again.

This includes:

1. Food tray carts
2. Trash/soiled linen carts
3. Surgical case carts

Other carts are washed in the cart washer on a scheduled basis:

1. Supply carts—monthly
2. Linen carts—monthly
3. Storage carts—semiannually or as needed
4. Miscellaneous carts—semiannually or as needed

When the cart washer is not operating properly, the steam gun will be used to clean carts and casters.

<u>Operating instructions:</u>

See equipment operating instruction manual.

Affected Departments

Reviewed _____

Subject	Effective Date 1-90	Latest Revision & Date
OPERATING THE VAC/STEAM STERILIZER		

The vac/steam sterilizer is used to terminally sterilize all hard goods (non-heat or moisture sensitive).

<u>Operating instructions:</u>

See equipment operating instruction manual.

If sterilizer is not operating properly, contact the manager or the maintenance department.

Affected Departments

Reviewed _____

Subject OPERATING THE STEAM STERILIZER (GRAVITY TYPE)	Effective Date 1-90	Latest Revision & Date

Standard time for exposure at 250°F:

Surgical packs in muslin wrappers—30 minutes
Utensils in muslin wrappers—15 to 30 minutes
Instruments in trays with muslin wrappers—15 to 30 minutes
Treatment trays (all kinds)—30 minutes
Solutions in Pyrex flasks—30 to 45 minutes

Operating instructions:

See equipment operating instruction manual.

Affected Departments

Reviewed _____

Subject	Effective Date	Latest Revision & Date
OPERATING THE ETO GAS STERILIZER	1-90	

The ETO gas sterilizer is used <u>only</u> to sterilize <u>heat- or moisture-sensitive</u> items. All items that can withstand the steam sterilizer should be sterilized by that method. If there is any question, contact the manager. Care must be exercised to avoid direct contact with the ETO agent.

<u>Operating instructions:</u>

See equipment operating instruction manual.

If the sterilizer is not operating properly, contact the manager or the maintenance department.

NOTE: Caution must be exercised when operating the equipment so that personnel are not exposed to excessive amounts of ETO. If exposure occurs, contact the manager and the safety officer of the institution and refer to the procedures in the safety manual.

Affected Departments

Reviewed _____

Subject	Effective Date	Latest Revision & Date
OPERATING THE ETO GAS AERATOR	1-90	

Items sterilized in an ETO gas sterilizer must be aerated before being issued for use, unless they are made of impervious products, such as solid stainless steel.

Consult the aeration chamber time schedule to determine the time required to effectively remove all residual ETO gas from the sterilized goods.

Operating instructions:

See equipment operating instruction manual.

If the aerator is not operating properly, contact the manager or the maintenance department.

Affected Departments

Reviewed _____

Subject	Effective Date 1-90	Latest Revision & Date
GAS STERILIZER LOG		

The gas sterilizer log is filled in whenever the sterilizer is used. (See sample.) It supplements the sterilizer load card records.

This log provides a permanent record of all items processed, time required, and operator involved.

The log is filed and maintained for seven (7) years. It is used for reference when problems or volume of activity need evaluation.

Affected Departments

Reviewed _____

Page 1 of 1

GAS STERILIZER LOG

DATE	CYCLE				LOAD #	LOAD CONTENTS: (ITEM(S)—DEPTS)	TECHNICIAN'S SIGNATURE	AERATOR CYCLE			
	TIME		HOT 140°F (2 hrs)	COLD 85°F (4½ hrs)				TIME		UNIT 1	UNIT 2
	IN	OUT						IN	OUT		

Subject		Effective Date 1-90	Latest Revision & Date
OPERATION AND USE OF WATER STILL			

The water still—model C—is an automatically controlled unit.

<u>Operating instructions:</u>

1. To start, open "water supply valve" and, after three (3) minutes, open "steam valve." The water can be used while the still is running.

2. When the water gauge appears filled, turn off both the steam valve and, then, the water valve.

3. Fill Pyrex flasks, write date on autoclave tape, and place tape on the flask ready for sterilization.

    For normal saline solution (sodium chloride):

    2,000ml distilled water
    8 sodium chloride tablets (2.25g each tablet)

    1,000ml distilled water
    4 sodium chloride tablets (2.25g each tablet)

4. Label flasks "normal saline."

5. <u>The still is to be cleaned by maintenance once a week to ensure that it works properly.</u>

Affected Departments

Reviewed _____

Subject		Effective Date 1-90	Latest Revision & Date
INSTRUMENT PROCESSING IN SURGERY			

Certain categories of instruments are <u>not</u> processed in materials management/processing. These are identified by the operating room supervisor. Some of them are:

1. Surgeon's own instruments (as specified)
2. Delicate eye instruments
3. Delicate ear instruments
4. Delicate fiberoptic equipment
5. Other delicate, special handling, or single quantity items so determined

Surgery will have two (2) <u>flash</u> sterilizers available for emergencies and for decontaminating surgeon's instruments before transport to another healthcare institution. Flash sterilizers will not be used for routine or terminal sterilizing.

All <u>terminal</u> sterilization will take place in materials management/processing.

Affected Departments

Reviewed _____

Subject	Effective Date	Latest Revision & Date
INSTRUMENT IDENTIFICATION	1-90	

All instruments will be etched (not engraved) with the hospital's initials, the month/year, and the initials of the department (materials management, operating room, etc.).

Color-coded tape will be used only for instruments owned by private surgeons.

Instruments will be processed in complete sets only. The set will be identified with a stainless steel tag showing the name and the number of that particular set on it. The tag will be permanently attached to the instrument tray/pan.

Affected Departments

Reviewed _____

Subject	Effective Date	Latest Revision & Date
INSTRUMENT INSPECTION/REPAIR/REPLACEMENT	1-90	

All instruments are processed in sets.

Operating room personnel discovering a defective instrument should tag it and leave it with the set.

On arrival in materials management/decontamination, the entire set will be processed. When the cycle is completed, the processing technician setting up surgical instruments will inspect all instruments and will remove malfunctioning ones (and the ones already labeled by operating room personnel).

All malfunctioning instruments that are removed are replaced with backup instruments from the pegboard or the backup cabinet when necessary. The technician will list which instruments were replaced in which set and keep the list with the Kardex file. A copy of the list is forwarded with the instruments to the operating room supervisor at least once each week. The operating room supervisor will then send them out for repair or order replacements.

When repaired or replacement instruments arrive, they are sent to surgery, then forwarded to materials management, processed, and placed in "backup."

Affected Departments

Reviewed _____

Page 1 of 1

Subject	Effective Date 1-90	Latest Revision & Date
SURGICAL INSTRUMENT PROCESSING		

1. After instruments and case carts have been used in surgery, they are to be taken to the soiled hold room. The surgical supply technician will empty suction bottles and other equipment and see that the used instruments are in a distilled water solution to keep soil and blood from drying/hardening on the instruments.

2. Case carts must be sent to decontamination right after each use.

3. As much as possible, each set is to be kept together for easy identification. There also will be an identification tag with each set.

4. Instruments are costly and are to be handled with care at all times. They should not be thrown into pans or dropped on top of other instruments.

5. Personnel taking care of the instruments must protect themselves by wearing gloves and the proper clothing for decontamination.

6. The instruments will be taken from the basin, rinsed, assembled on the U-shaped racks, and placed in the instrument pans marked from that set. All points are to be up so as not to ruin the instrument, the pan, or the machine. Longer instruments, such as retractors, ring forceps, and long knife handles, will be put alongside the instrument pan in a horizontal position.

7. Two instrument pans will fit into one washer/sterilizer basket for washing. They should be set down firmly on the bottom, no higher than 15 inches from the bottom of the machine.

Affected Departments

Reviewed _____

Subject	Effective Date 1-90	Latest Revision & Date
INSTRUMENT MILKING		

All instruments processed are "milked" after each cleaning to lubricate moving parts and prevent corrosion.

1. To prepare milk solution, mix one gallon of instrument milk with six gallons of water, or according to the manufacturer's specifications.

   The milk should be changed as often as necessary, but at least once a week. Microbiology cultures of the solution will be taken periodically.

2. Submerge the basket of cleaned instruments into the instrument milk. Let stand for one (1) minute.

3. Stiff instruments should soak for at least one (1) hour or overnight.

4. When removing the instruments from the instrument milk bath, drain thoroughly over the milk pan. <u>Do not dry the instruments.</u>

5. Remove the instruments from the basket and transport to work area for assembling.

6. Excessive milking can cause "slippery" instruments. Check them carefully before and after milking to avoid this.

Affected Departments

Reviewed _____

Page 1 of 1

Subject		Effective Date 1-90	Latest Revision & Date
INSTRUMENT INSPECTION			

After the instruments come out of a completed washer/sterilizer cycle:

1. Examine each instrument for cleanliness.

2. Return instruments that are not clean to decontamination.

3. Inspect hinged instruments (clamps and forceps) for any stiffness and for proper alignment of jaws and teeth. Joints should move smoothly. Jaws and teeth should meet perfectly. Ratchets should close easily and hold firmly.

4. Inspect the edges of sharp and semisharp instruments (scissors, curettes) for chips, dents, or dull spots. If any of the above are found, the instrument must be repaired.

5. Examine plated instruments for chips, sharp edges, or worn spots. Blood and tissue could stick to chipped plating. Sharp edges could damage tissue and rubber gloves. Worn spots could rust.

6. Inspect malleable instruments (probes and retractors) for dents and bends. Bent instruments are difficult for the physician to mold to the patient. Malleable instruments should be flat and smooth.

7. Hold any instrument in poor working condition for repair. Instruments should be repaired at the first sign of damage. Surgery is not the only department that can determine when an instrument needs repair. It can be noted in processing. Instruments in poor condition are a handicap to the surgeon and a hazard to the patient.

8. Separate the basic instruments from special instruments. Basic instruments are those used in the major or minor, plastic, or vaginal sets, etc. Special instruments are those that are wrapped separately, such as gall bladder and thoracic.

9. Disassemble instruments with movable parts (do not separate forceps), but keep all parts together so they can be easily reassembled. Steam cannot contact the unexposed parts of assembled instruments.

10. Leave all box locks open for sterilization. The sterilizing agent must contact all surfaces to ensure sterilization.

11. Consult the Kardex file and assemble the trays using the correct number and type of instruments. <u>Do not substitute</u> one instrument for another.

12. Place heavy instruments on the bottom of the tray, delicate on top, and retractors above or to one side.

Affected Departments

Reviewed _____

Subject	Effective Date	Latest Revision & Date
INSTRUMENT TRAY ASSEMBLY	1-90	

Instrument and procedural trays are to be assembled in a manner that provides for both penetration of the sterilizing agent (steam or ETO) and for ease of use.

The Kardex file and corresponding photograph are to be used to ensure the proper setup of all trays. The reference catalog should be used to identify any instrument when necessary.

After assembly, the trays are to be wrapped in a double thickness of nonwoven paper (or two double muslin wraps), labeled fully, initialed, and set aside for sterilizing.

Consult Procedure #14.2 for proper labeling, wrapping, and shelf life of all trays.

Affected Departments

Reviewed _____

Page 1 of 1

Subject	Effective Date	Latest Revision & Date
PROCESSING NEEDLES	1-90	

Generally, disposable surgical needles will be used on surgical trays.

Reusable surgical needles will be hand-processed by surgery in the surgery cleanup area. When materials management cleans needles, the following procedure is followed:

1. Take precautions for contamination: use gloves, masks, etc.

2. Carefully remove needle from tray and carry to work area.

3. Take needle apart and rinse thoroughly.

4. Clean needle with warm soapy water and shoot solution through the lumen of the needle.

5. Clean the hub and all threaded parts with cotton-tip applicator.

6. Rinse needle thoroughly.

7. Inspect needle; if it is not clean, return it to decontamination.

8. Rinse needle again and follow up with cotton-tip applicator.

9. If needle is clean, place with extra parts (stylet, etc.) into a needle basket.

10. Close the needle basket and place into a washer basket with other articles to be processed.

11. Place the loaded basket onto the conveyer belt for processing through the washer/sterilizer.

Affected Departments

Reviewed _____

Subject		Effective Date 1-90	Latest Revision & Date
	LABORATORY GLASS CLEANING		

The laboratory cleans all the glassware items it uses in its own automatic glassware washer.

Any laboratory glassware sent to decontamination should be wrapped in a plastic bag and sent to the laboratory for processing.

Affected Departments

Reviewed _____

Subject	Effective Date	Latest Revision & Date
PROCESSING SYRINGES	1-90	

To process syringes:

1. Separate barrel and plunger.

2. Thoroughly rinse items under running water at a work station sink.

3. Place the syringe into a test tube basket.

4. Load syringe basket into the washer/sterilizer.

5. If the washer/sterilizer is being used, wash syringes in the sonic washer.

6. Rinse with distilled water.

7. Route syringe final assembly and processing.

Affected Departments

Reviewed _____

Subject	Effective Date	Latest Revision & Date
PROCESSING PUMP EQUIPMENT	1-90	

To process pump equipment, refer to the manufacturer's operating and cleaning instructions. Then, take the following steps:

1. Remove all disposable tubing and deposit in a wastebasket.

2. Remove suction bottles and caps for separate processing.

3. If overflow bottle has been used during patient care, it should be removed and reprocessed.

4. Clean pump by wiping with a cloth and detergent solution. Start at the top and wipe downward.

5. Using another cloth and tap water, remove the soapy film. Again, start at the top and work downward.

6. Dry the pump with a clean towel.

7. Routinely clean and oil the wheels on Emerson and Wangensteen units.

8. Transport pumps through the door to the clean section.

Once on the clean side:

1. Reassemble pumps at work station.

    a. Inspect pump for cleanliness.

    b. Reassemble the pump so that the shorter stem of the metal tubing is connected to the rubber tubing of the pump and the longer stem of the metal tubing is connected to the Harris flush tubing.

    c. Attach $1/4$-inch connectors to the end of the Harris flush tubing.

2. Test the pumps for proper operation.

    a. Check the electrical plug and wiring for frayed or loose wires.

    b. Plug the pump's electrical cord into an electrical wall outlet.

    c. Test machines with suction collar switch set at both high and low intensities.

    d. Flip the "on-off" button to "on."

    e. A red pilot light will come on.

    f. Inspect the jar lid and tubing for a proper, tight fit.

Affected Departments

Reviewed _____

Subject		Effective Date 1-90	Latest Revision & Date
PROCESSING PUMP EQUIPMENT (cont.)			

g. The red pilot light will go off.

h. Observe the clear, plastic tubing attached to the jar.

i. If tap water is suctioned through the tube, the pump is operational.

j. Secure the plastic tubing on the side of the machine.

k. Switch the suction collar button to "low."

l. Unplug, rewind, and fasten the electrical cord to the machine.

3. Place a section of tape on the pump.

4. Record the date and initial the tape.

5. Cover the pump with a plastic cover.

6. Transport the pump to the storage area.

7. Notify the manager of any pumps that have mechanical failure. A work order will be completed, and the pump will be transported to the maintenance department.

8. Record in the equipment repair log the pump's serial number, description of the mechanical problem, and the date.

9. When the pump is returned, test it again for proper operation.

10. Place a check mark (✓) in the equipment repair log.

Subject	Effective Date	Latest Revision & Date
PROCESSING SUCTION BOTTLE UNITS	1-90	

To process suction bottle units, refer to the manufacturer's operating and cleaning instructions. Then, take the following steps:

1. Suction bottles

   a. Remove tops at a work station sink.

   b. Rinse bottles and tops under running water at a work station sink.

   c. Place items in a washer basket.

   d. Place the loaded basket onto the conveyor belt for processing through the washer/sterilizer.

2. Suction bottle tops

   a. Wash bottle tops at a work station sink using a brush and soapy solution.

   b. Wash the plastic rims with a scrub brush and soapy solution.

   c. Rinse the bottle tops with running water.

   d. Place bottle tops in a washer/sterilizer basket.

   e. Place the loaded basket onto the conveyor belt for processing through the washer/sterilizer.

   f. Discard worn suction bottle tops or those that do not properly seal and replace them with new suction bottle tops.

3. Suction bottle storage

   a. Reassemble suction bottles.

   b. Cover suction bottles with a dust cover.

   c. Transport suction bottles to the storage area.

Affected Departments

Reviewed _____

Page 1 of 1

Subject	Effective Date	Latest Revision & Date
PROCESSING RESPIRATORY THERAPY EQUIPMENT	1-90	

1. Respiratory therapy equipment is sent to decontamination via the soiled cart lift in the soiled hold room.

2. Machines that remain on the various floors/areas are disassembled by respiratory therapy personnel. The parts to be sent to decontamination are placed in a tote box marked "respiratory therapy," located in the soiled hold room.

3. Respiratory therapy personnel wipe down the machines that will remain on the floors/areas with disinfectant and return them to the holding area.

4. After processing, items are returned to respiratory therapy by dispatch personnel.

5. For procedures on care and handling of specific equipment, see the "respiratory therapy" section of the Kardex file or the equipment manufacturer's instructions for operating and cleaning the equipment.

Items processed for respiratory therapy include:

1. Air Viva bag

2. Hope II bag

3. Bourns respirometer tube

4. Bennett mouth seal

5. Bird adult Q

6. Bird pediatric Q

7. CAM tubing and bag

8. HV-11

9. HV-12 CAM nebulizer

10. Bendix ultrasonic

11. DeVilbiss continuous feed

12. DeVilbiss ultrasonic setup

13. Mistogen continuous feed

14. Mistogen ultrasonic setup

Affected Departments

Reviewed _____

Subject	Effective Date	Latest Revision & Date
PROCESSING RESPIRATORY THERAPHY EQUIPMENT (cont.)	1-90	

15. Hudson analyzer "T"

16. MA-1 cascade

17. MA-1 drain

18. MA-1 filter kit

19. MA-1 ped circuit

20. MA-1 spirometer

21. Noseclips

22. Oxygen humidifier

23. One-way valve

24. Mask

25. Room humidifier (wash only)

26. Incentive spirometer (gas only)

Affected Departments

Reviewed _____

Subject	Effective Date 1-90	Latest Revision & Date
PROCESSING RUBBER CATHETERS		

A limited number of rubber catheters are purchased unsterile and sterilized by the institution before use. Catheters are <u>not</u> reused.

To process rubber catheters:

1. Collect and group catheters at work table.

2. Inspect catheters for damage and cleanliness.

3. If catheters are being prepared for steam sterilization, rinse the catheters with distilled water.

4. Using a syringe, shoot distilled water through the lumen. Steam will not pass through the lumen unless it is wet.

5. Place the catheter in a long peel-pack sterilization pouch.

6. Label the pouch (include make and size of catheter, date, and operator's initials).

7. If catheters are being prepared for gas sterilization, the catheters must be completely dry. Gas sterilization is recommended because it is less harmful to the rubber than steam. Proper aeration time must follow gas sterilization.

8. Transport the catheters to the appropriate sterilizer.

9. Return sterilized catheters to the sterile stores area.

Affected Departments

Reviewed _____

Subject	Effective Date	Latest Revision & Date
PROCESSING RUBBER/PLASTIC TUBING	1-90	

To process rubber/plastic tubing:

1. Make sure all tubing is clean and free of debris.

2. If rubber/plastic tubing is being prepared for steam sterilization, rinse the tubing with distilled water.

3. Using a syringe, shoot distilled water through the lumen. Steam will not pass through the lumen unless it is wet.

4. If the tubing is being prepared for gas sterilization, the tubing must be dry.

5. Pack tubing in a sterilization pouch.

6. Attach a label showing date and operator's initials on the outer wrapper.

7. Transport tubing to the sterilizer.

8. Return sterilized plastic tubing to the sterile stores area.

Affected Departments

Reviewed _____

Subject	Effective Date 1-90	Latest Revision & Date
PROCESSING BASINS		

To process basins:

1. Empty basins of any contents.

2. Rinse basins under running water at a work station sink.

3. Place basins in a washer/sterilizer basket rack.

4. Place loaded basket rack onto the conveyor belt for processing through the washer/sterilizer.

5. If terminal sterilization is required, wrap basins using the double-wrapper technique.

Affected Departments

Reviewed _____

Subject	Effective Date	Latest Revision & Date
PROCESSING REUSABLE UTENSILS	1-90	

To process reusable utensils:

1. Empty utensils of any contents.

2. Rinse utensils under running water at a work station sink.

3. Place utensils on a washer/sterilizer rack.

4. Place loaded rack onto the conveyor belt for transport to the washer/sterilizer.

5. Process the utensil load through the washer/sterilizer.

6. Inspect the contents after processing. If any dirt remains, reprocess immediately.

7. If terminal sterilization is required, wrap utensils using the double-wrapper technique.

Affected Departments

Reviewed _____

Subject		Effective Date 1-90	Latest Revision & Date
PROCESSING ASEPTO SYRINGES			

Where possible, disposable Asepto syringes will be used.

To process reusable Asepto syringes:

1. Assemble the Asepto syringe and correct rubber bulb.

2. Make sure the Asepto syringe is clean and clear of any obstruction by filling the syringe with distilled water.

3. Disassemble the rubber bulb and Asepto syringe for proper sterilization.

4. Wrap Asepto syringe in gauze to prevent breakage.

5. Place Asepto syringe into sterilization pouch.

6. Attach a label showing date and operator's initials.

7. Transport the Asepto syringe to the steam sterilizer.

8. Return sterilized Asepto syringes to the sterile stores area.

Affected Departments

Reviewed _____

Subject	Effective Date 1-90	Latest Revision & Date
PROCESSING PATIENT CARE EQUIPMENT		

To process patient care equipment, refer to the manufacturer's instructions for proper operation and cleaning.

1. Oral suction machines:

   a. Thoroughly wash the machine with a disinfectant, rinse, and wipe dry so that metal parts will not rust. The metal airways and black rubber stopper are to be soaked for 15 minutes. After 15 minutes, rinse the items in distilled (sterile) water and reassemble the machine.

   b. Run the machine to ensure that it is in good working condition.

2. Gomco Levine suction (Wangensteen):

   Plug in and draw a soap solution through the system; wash all parts. Replace plastic suction tubing. Twice a year, change the small plastic tubing to the overflow bottles. Also, clean overflow bottle frequently. Reassemble.

3. Emerson pump:

   a. Plug in to test if gauge is working correctly. Remove all tubing and dispose of it. Wash all parts in a disinfectant and rinse thoroughly. Use a bottle brush to clean bottles. Reassemble, adding tubing, and ready machine for use.

   b. Place two sterile forceps, one 1,000ml sterile pitcher, and an entire package of tubing with the machine. Be sure to cover with 4 x 4 dressing and hold in place with a rubber band. Cover the entire machine with a plastic cover. Place a sterile green plug on the machine.

4. Thoracic pleural pump (Gomco):

   Wash the machine and extra parts in a disinfectant. Discard the plastic suction tubing, being careful not to discard the tubing inside the glass flask. Wrap the drainage bottle for sterilization and put it on the machine. Leave the tubing in the box.

5. K-Pad:

   Wash the machine and pad with a disinfectant and rinse. Empty the distilled water in the machine and clean the inside with applicators to remove the residue. Reassemble; fill machine with distilled water to water line, and set the temperature gauge to 95°. Check the temperature gauge again when delivering the machine.

Affected Departments

Reviewed _____

Page 1 of 2

Subject	Effective Date 1-90	Latest Revision & Date
PROCESSING PATIENT CARE EQUIPMENT (cont.)		

6. <u>K-Kooler:</u>

a. Check that all parts of the machine and pad have been returned. Wash the machine and pad with a disinfectant and rinse.

b. After the machine has been washed, rinsed, and dried, place a plastic cover over it and move to storage area.

7. <u>K-Thermia:</u>

a. Wash with a disinfectant; thoroughly clean the stand also. The thermometer section may be removed when taking the machine from the stand. Wash pads thoroughly and roll up; roll tubing around pads. Re-assemble.

b. Place the rectal probe, after washing, in the box and place on top of the machine along with a 1,000ml bottle of 40-percent alcohol. The instruction sheet should also be placed with the machine. Cover with a plastic cover.

8. <u>K-Thermette:</u>

Follow the same procedure as for the K-Thermia.

9. <u>Cradles:</u>

Wash the cradle in a disinfectant, rinse, and place in a plastic bag.

10. <u>Perineal light:</u>

When returned, wash the unit with a disinfectant, rinse, and dry. Check bulbs and store in a plastic bag.

Affected Departments

Reviewed _____

Subject		Effective Date	Latest Revision & Date
	CASE CART SYSTEM	1-90	

1. Ordering the case cart

A case cart requisition (see typical sample) is used by operating room personnel to order case carts from materials management/processing. The appropriate requisition should be used from a choice of major, minor, or neuro/ortho/vascular. The requisitions are sent to materials management as soon as they are ready so the case carts can be assembled. Operating room personnel prepare a case cart requisition for each surgical procedure to be performed, based on the surgical schedule and the surgeon's preference cards. Any extra quantities or special items needed should be noted in the blank spaces provided on the requisition.

Special attention must be paid to the time of the case and be so noted in the space provided. Any cases added on can be listed as "to follow."

The operating room personnel send requisitions for the first cases at 9A.M. and then send all remaining case cart requisitions to materials management/processing no later than 2P.M., the day before the procedures are scheduled, along with the surgical schedule for that day.

2. Setup of case carts

Case cart requisitions received from surgery are sorted in time-of-case sequence. All "first" cases are set up first (cases scheduled for 7A.M.). "To follow," or afternoon, cases are set up last.

The processing technician uses the case cart requisition like a grocery list, pulling all items ordered on the requisition from the shelves in sterile stores, and placing them on the case cart. Care must be taken to locate items on the cart so that they will fit properly and not be damaged.

The processing technician marks the quantities issued in the appropriate column of the requisition. If an item, or the ordered quantity of any item, is unavailable at the time the case cart is being set up, the processing technician circles the "quantity issued" in red. Later that shift or before the cart is sent to surgery, the items are obtained, placed on the cart, and the quantity-issued figure is adjusted. A copy of the case cart requisition is removed and retained in a file in materials management/processing in chronological order for thirty (30) days. This data base is used to address problems, to assess quality performance, and to make changes to requisitions based on usage.

The last copy of the three-part case cart requisition is attached to the case cart itself and accompanies it to surgery. It remains with the cart as a means of identification and is returned with the cart to the decontamination area of materials management after use.

Affected Departments

Reviewed _____

Subject		Effective Date 1-90	Latest Revision & Date
	CASE CART SYSTEM (cont.)		

OPERATING ROOM CASE CART REQUISITION — ABDOMINAL CASE

PROCEDURE _____ REQUESTED BY _____ DATE RECEIVED _____
SURGEON _____ DATE _____ FILLING TIME _____
PATIENT _____ TIME _____ FILLED BY _____
OPERATING ROOM # _____ TRANSPORT TIME _____

REQ.	REC'D	USED	ITEM #	LINEN		REQ.	REC'D	USED	STERILE WRAPPED SUPPLIES
—	—	—	72-48741	100 minor pack		—	—	—	ABD pads
—	—	—	72-65514	131 lap pack		—	—	—	Basin set
—	—	—	72-76583	410 lg. gown		—	—	—	Lap packs
—	—	—	72-76656	440 xlg. gown		—	—	—	Light handles
—	—	—	72-36212	8376 table cover		—	—	—	Medicine glass
—	—	—	72-32926	8355 sm. sheet		—	—	—	Prep pack
—	—	—	72-32837	8346 lg. sheet		—	—	—	Retractor covers
						—	—	—	Towels
				SURGEON GLOVES					
—	—	—	68-08212	Triflex size 6					**INSTRUMENTS**
—	—	—	68-08263	Triflex size 6½		—	—	—	Major set
—	—	—	68-08417	Triflex size 7		—	—	—	Minor set
—	—	—	68-08549	Triflex size 7½		—	—	—	Gall-bladder set
—	—	—	68-08689	Triflex size 8		—	—	—	Intestinal set
—	—	_____				—	—	_____	
—	—	_____				—	—	_____	
						—	—	—	Curved hemostats
				SUPPLIES		—	—	—	Deaver retractors
—	—	—	76-45155	Bulb syringe		—	—	—	Harrington retractors
—	—	—	84-12111	Bovie cord		—	—	—	Haneys
—	—	—	84-54027	Bovie plate, disp		—	—	—	Kochers
—	—	—	71-07382	Foam head rest		—	—	—	Long rt.-angle clamps
—	—	—	72-70429	Incise drape-3M		—	—	—	Long needle holder
—	—	—	84-54043	K-dissectors		—	—	—	Ribbon retractor
—	—	—	66-61971	Sponge, x-ray 4 x 4		—	—	—	Spring retractors
—	—	—	66-23573	Sponge, dressing 4 x 4		—	—	—	Towel clips
—	—	—	84-39621	Suction canister		—	—	—	Vanderbilts
—	—	—	78-05799	Tube, cond. sterile					
—	—	—	84-00229	Urine meter					**SOLUTIONS**
—	—	—	84-17615	VI-drape 7"		—	—	—	61-00104 1500 normal saline
—	—	—	84-17622	VI-drape 9"		—	—	—	61-00066 1500 sterile water
—	—	—	84-99748	VI-drape, surgical film		—	—	_____	
						—	—	_____	
									OTHER
						—	—	_____	
						—	—	_____	

Affected Departments

Reviewed _____

Subject	Effective Date	Latest Revision & Date
CASE CART SYSTEM (cont.)	1-90	

3. Dispatch of case carts

   Prepared case carts are sent to surgery the evening before the scheduled day. At 7:30P.M., the processing technician calls surgery and informs operating room personnel that it is time to send up the case carts.

   The first two cases of the day are then sent up on the clean operating room cart lift. Operating room personnel place these carts at the door of the room in which the procedure will take place the next day. The carts should be inspected at that time so that any errors can be detected and corrected immediately. Any problems and the corrective action taken must be so noted on the requisition. (Use reverse side if necessary.)

   All later-day and "to follow" case carts are sent up to surgery via the cart lift at 7A.M. the next day or as scheduled. These carts are received by operating room personnel.

4. Use of the case cart

   When the procedure is about to begin, the case cart is moved into the operating room, "opened up," and used as a back table during the procedure.

   Operating room personnel must take care that unused items do not come into contact with the patient or any used items; since clean unused items will be returned for reuse without being processed.

   The unused clean items are separated and placed on a utility cart in the clean corridor for return to materials management via the clean cart lift. The supply technician in surgery sends these to materials management when the cart is full or at the end of the shift.

5. Supply charges

   All supply items sent to surgery are charged to surgery via the case cart requisition. Surgery is responsible for charging the patient, when appropriate, using the code numbers on the requisition.

Affected Departments

Reviewed _____

Subject		Effective Date	Latest Revision & Date
CASE CART SYSTEM (cont.)		1-90	

6. <u>Backup supplies</u>

The operating room has carts in the sterile corridor that contain a variety of items that may be required <u>in addition to</u> those on the case cart. Items are taken from these carts by operating room personnel to be used during the surgical procedures. Unused items should be placed back on the carts in their appropriate locations.

The carts are: (1) suture, (2) IV fluid, (3) irrigation fluid, (4) med/surg, and (5) instruments. These carts are restocked <u>daily</u> by materials management. The supply technician obtains the supplies from materials management, Monday through Friday, at 7A.M. and, if necessary, at 3P.M. Items needed during a case and not found on the backup carts are obtained via a telephone call to sterile stores. The processing technician obtains the item and sends it to surgery via the clean cart lift on a spare cart or in a tote box. The item(s) requested and sent is noted on the materials management log. Items called for regularly are added to the case cart or backup carts.

A limited number (and quantity) of surgical supplies are stored in the operating rooms. These include items that cannot be anticipated on the case cart requisition and for which surgery staff should not leave the room once the procedure has started. These items are restocked daily by surgery personnel.

7. <u>Cart return</u>

After the operating procedure is completed, the operating room personnel:

a. Sort all unused, clean items and place them in the clean corridor on a clean cart. The supply technician (if available) calls materials management/processing to arrange for all clean items to be returned via the clean cart lift. These items should be returned by 3:30P.M., Monday through Friday, or as the cart becomes full.

b. Bag all linen and trash (green bag for linen, buff-color bag for trash).

c. Place used/soiled instruments (box locks <u>open</u>) in the distilled water in the pan or in a basin and place on the middle shelf of the case cart.

d. Place all other returnable (for reprocessing) items on the other shelves of the case cart.

e. Return a copy of the requisition with the case cart.

f. <u>Cover</u> the case cart with the cover provided.

Affected Departments

Reviewed _____

Subject	Effective Date	Latest Revision & Date
CASE CART SYSTEM (cont.)	1-90	

g. Place trash and linen bags or hampers in the soiled hold room (or the operating room). The linen and trash generated from that procedure is put in a convertible trash cart that is used to hold (transport) the bags. The soiled cart is taken to the soiled utility room by housekeeping personnel.

h. Prepare the soiled cart and take it to the soiled utility room or contact the supply technician to do so. The linen is placed in the linen chute/tube station, and the trash is placed in the trash chute/tube for dissemination. The covered soiled case cart is lined up in front of the soiled cart lift and sent to materials management/decontamination.

8. <u>Emergency case carts</u>

One emergency case cart is set up and maintained in materials management to be used only in emergencies. To obtain the emergency case cart, call materials management/processing, operating room personnel, or the nursing supervisor to notify materials management that a cart is to be sent up. (Call dispatch if needed between 11P.M. and 7A.M.) Follow with the appropriate case cart requisition. Materials management personnel will give this request <u>top priority</u> and send it to the operating room via the clean cart lift. Materials management will assemble another emergency case cart immediately after verification that the one sent has been put to use.

Items on the emergency case cart are <u>never</u> used for routine purposes. The cart is checked at least weekly by the processing technician assigned to that area for outdated or missing items.

The cart is labeled "emergency" and is stored covered in sterile stores.

9. <u>Supply cost allocation</u>

Most stock supply items used by surgery are stored and managed by materials management. These are <u>charged to the surgery department</u> when the case cart requisition is filled.

Certain nonstock items stored in surgery are managed by operating room personnel. They are ordered through the purchasing office either on a nonstock request for purchasing services form or on a traveling requisition card. The supply technician assigned to surgery assists with the handling of these items as needed.

10. <u>Implants and prosthetic devices</u>

Some of these items are stored in materials management and are ordered as used/needed by materials management personnel on a traveling requisition card. Surgery is charged for these items as used. Total hip parts and other devices are ordered and stored by surgery.

Affected Departments

Reviewed _____

Page 5 of 6

Subject	Effective Date	Latest Revision & Date
CASE CART SYSTEM (cont.)	1-90	

11. Special supply/equipment items

Surgery may require a specialty item not carried by the institution. When this occurs, operating room personnel notify materials management, in writing, that such an item is needed and state specifically what is needed (size, catalog number, etc.). Materials management orders it and forwards it to the operating room when it arrives.

Affected Departments

Reviewed _____

Subject	Effective Date	Latest Revision & Date
PROCESSING TRACTION EQUIPMENT	1-90	

To process traction equipment:

1. Remove traction sash cords.

2. Wash items with cloth, warm water, and detergent.

3. Rinse with clean cloth and tap water.

4. Dry items with clean towel.

5. Steam sterilize items using the proper technique.

Affected Departments

Reviewed _____

Subject	Effective Date 1-90	Latest Revision & Date
PROCESSING INFECTIOUS, HAZARDOUS MATERIALS		

The institution's infection control committee has established policies and procedures for dealing with highly infectious and hazardous materials used in the care of patients afflicted with diseases such as acquired immune deficiency syndrome (AIDS) and other conditions that require patients to be placed in isolation.

These policies and procedures are designed to protect patients, staff, visitors, and the community. These regulations meet or exceed those developed by the city, state, and federal health authorities.

Staff are instructed to refer and adhere to these policies and procedures, which can be found in the infection control manual—material processing section.

Affected Departments

Reviewed _____

Subject	Effective Date 1-90	Latest Revision & Date
STERILIZING FOR OTHER INSTITUTIONS AND PHYSICIANS		

In an emergency, such as when another facility's or physician's own sterilizer fails to operate, the hospital may provide sterilizing services for them. All such requests must be authorized by the director <u>before</u> providing the service.

Requests from other parties for reprocessing/sterilization services should be submitted in writing to the director for review and should include a list of all items and quantities that must be sterilized.

If authorization is provided, all items are to be sterilized for these parties <u>after</u> the hospital's own demands have been met and time is available in the sterilizer. The hospital does <u>not</u> interrupt its own sterilizing schedule. These outside requests have a secondary priority.

The items presented are to be wrapped according to proper, accepted procedures and labeled. Special handling/processing directions should also be included.

NOTE: In <u>all</u> instances, the institution will follow its own policies and procedures for proper handling, packaging, and sterilization of items from other parties. Items not conforming to these practices will not be accepted.

The hospital assumes no liability for condition or use of the items after they have been processed.

The hospital may, in a similar situation, send its own items to another facility for sterilization. The same conditions apply, and the same procedure is to be followed.

Affected Departments

Reviewed _____

Department   MATERIALS MANAGEMENT
     Policy/
Procedure #14.34

Subject	Effective Date	Latest Revision & Date
PREPARATION OF EXTERNAL SOLUTIONS/FLUIDS	1-90	

When economically desirable or if the availability of a purchased product is problematic, the hospital may produce sterile irrigation and related solutions used for <u>external</u> treatments only. Using the sterile-flask technique, the hospital provides a quality product that, when administered to the patient, is safe and cost effective.

1. Empty any remaining solution from flask. Remove and discard date tag from flask.

2. Place flask in designated holding area in the decontamination area.

         Used flasks should be confined to the soiled area.

3. Hold flasks in collection area and transfer at predetermined intervals.

         Carts facilitate handling and transfer.

<u>Cleaning flasks (manual method):</u>

         <u>Special instructions:</u>

1. Rinse each flask with hot tap water.

         Remove any residue of solution.

2. Wash each flask in hot water containing a properly diluted germicide. Follow the directions on the label.

         Detergent or germicide should be free-rinsing.

3. Use a long-handled brush to scrub inside the flask.

         Nylon brush should be used.

4. Rinse thoroughly with tap water.

         Rinsing should include heavy use of water.

5. Rinse thoroughly with distilled water.

6. Inspect each flask for "water breaks" and for damage; rewash unclean flasks; discard damaged flasks.

         Chipped or cracked flasks should not be used.

7. Place on drain cart in the inverted position.

         Inverted position allows final rinse water to drain; provides less chance of dust or other foreign particles settling on the mouth or inside flask.

8. Transfer drainage cart to filling area.

         Flasks are ready for use.

9. Repeat distilled-water rinse if not filled within four (4) hours.

         Remove any foreign particles that might have collected during the holding period.

Affected Departments

Reviewed _____

Subject	Effective Date	Latest Revision & Date
PREPARATION OF EXTERNAL SOLUTIONS/FLUIDS (cont.)	1-90	

Preparation of distilled water:

1. Use only freshly distilled water. Allow one (1) quart to drain off before filling solution flasks.

2. Clean spigot with a 70-percent alcohol sponge before draining water.

3. Fill flasks from the spigot. Be sure to fill the flask to the proper level marked on each flask.

4. Apply identification label.

5. Date each flask; place date the flask was autoclaved on the single-use label.

6. Apply preassembled, reuseable cap and collar.

7. Be sure all flasks are clearly marked — STERILE DISTILLED WATER.

Special instructions:

Purity of water used should equal that for parenteral solutions.

At best, under the most careful regulation of the exhaust, there will be a loss of 3 to 5 percent of fluid by vaporization.

Ensure effective rotation of flask during storage. The vacuum-seal use maintains sterility indefinitely.

Assembled unit is easier to apply; less chance of faulty closure.

Sterilization of solutions:

1. Sterilize solutions as soon as preparation and flasking have been completed.

2. Exposure periods at 250° to 254°F:
   75-250ml—20 minutes
   500-1,000ml—30 minutes
   1,500-2,000ml—40 minutes

3. Remove the load from the sterilizer after completion of cycle or when chamber pressure gauge registers zero.

4. Cool to room temperature and check each flask for vacuum seal by lightly striking the top or bottom of the flask with the heel of the hand; a distinctive click (known as water hammer) should be heard.

Affected Departments

Reviewed _____

Subject	Effective Date	Latest Revision & Date
PREPARATION OF EXTERNAL SOLUTIONS/FLUIDS (cont.)	1-90	

General principles:

1. Once each month, the water in the still holding tank is to be cultured. Reports received from the laboratory are kept on file in processing. Positive cultures should be investigated immediately. No further production of solutions will continue until the problem is identified and solved.

2. Sterile water samples are to be tested by the laboratory each month, with a written report kept on file in processing.

3. The first 500ml of distillate at the beginning of each day's operation is to be discarded.

4. Reclaimed flasks or bottles, such as commercial IV solution bottles, should never be used to prepare solutions.

Preparation of normal saline solution (sodium chloride):

    2,000ml distilled water
    8 sodium chloride tablets (2.25g each tablet)

    1,000ml distilled water
    4 sodium chloride tablets (2.25g each tablet)

1. Flasks should be labeled "normal saline."

2. The still is to be cleaned by maintenance once a week to ensure that it works properly.

Subject	Effective Date 1-90	Latest Revision & Date
REQUESTS FOR CHANGES IN PROCEDURAL TRAY COMPONENTS		

Materials management maintains a current file listing the components of all procedural trays and setups of equipment.

The tray components and files are changed to reflect the current needs of the user departments as the changes occur. They are reviewed at least annually and updated as needed.

Changes are made on the tray and in the file only after the following procedure has been completed:

1. The request for the change is put in writing and submitted to the nursing supervisor (clinical care coordinator) of the affected area.

2. The request is forwarded to the director of nursing for review. If the impact of the change is substantial, she or he will forward it to the chief of staff/surgery for review before presenting the request to the appropriate committee of physicians or surgeons for additional review.

3. The committee chairperson or chief of the department will approve/authorize the change with a signature.

4. The authorization is returned to nursing, copied, and forwarded to the materials management processing manager.

5. Materials management makes the correction on the file, makes copies for those requiring them, and makes the change on the tray or setup.

Any expenses caused by the change are charged to the user department.

Affected Departments

Reviewed _____

Subject	Effective Date 1-90	Latest Revision & Date
WRAPPING MATERIALS		

The selection of the appropriate wrapper depends on the type and size of item to be sterilized, the necessary shelf life, and ease of opening required by the user.

Subject	Effective Date	Latest Revision & Date
STERILIZER BREAKDOWN	1-90	

In the event of a sterilizer malfunction or aborted cycle, notify the following:

1. Maintenance (will determine if its personnel can repair the equipment or if the manufacturer's service technician must be contacted)

2. The material processing manager

3. The purchasing department (its personnel may call the manufacturer's service technician)

4. The nursing service supervisor

5. Any departments requiring items to be sterilized (steam or ETO gas) (e.g., surgery, respiratory therapy, cardiac catheterization laboratory)

   When notifying the other departments involved, explain what steps have already been taken (contact of sales or service representative, maintenance, etc.) and what length of time the service is likely to be interrupted.

Processing personnel will call the manufacturer's service technician's office, home, or answering service, as necessary, if a breakdown occurs after hours.

When calling:

1. Give specific information regarding exactly what happened.

2. Obtain the time the repair technician will be on site to correct the situation. If unable to contact the repair technician, call the sales representative at office or home and ask for assistance. State that immediate response is critical. Keep trying until verbal contact is made with either party.

If an item(s) is locked in the sterilizer and must be made available before repairs can be made, maintenance may be able to release the item(s) from the sterilizer.

If such an interruption continues for 24 hours or more, another hospital may be contacted by the processing manager to arrange for the sterilizing of items until the equipment is repaired.

Affected Departments

Reviewed _____

Subject	Effective Date 1-90	Latest Revision & Date
CHEMICAL PROCESSING		

Instruments and utensils that cannot be terminally sterilized and that do not come into contact with patients' tissue via body cavities or surgical sites must be sanitized or disinfected between patient uses.

The infection control committee establishes all guidelines, procedures, and acceptable chemicals and methods to be used to render items safe for use.

Generally, all items are thoroughly cleaned before use. When chemical products are used, the manufacturer's procedures will be followed. Any deviations are reviewed by the infection control committee in conjunction with the processing manager.

Affected Departments

Reviewed _____

Subject	Effective Date	Latest Revision & Date
CLEANING OF PROCESSING EQUIPMENT	1-90	

1. <u>Steam sterilizers</u>

   a. <u>Daily</u>:

   The plug screen strainer is to be removed, and lint and sediment are to be cleaned from the pores with a brush.

   b. <u>Weekly</u>:

   The inside of the chamber is to be washed every Saturday night. Sterilizers are to be turned off at 11P.M. for cool down so that the day shift can clean. Calgonite is the cleaning solution (follow manufacturer's instructions) to be applied with a long-handled cellulose sponge mop. After cleaning, the sterilizer must be rinsed thoroughly.

   The plug screen should be removed, and the chamber drain line flushed with hot solution of trisodium phosphate (one ounce to one quart of water). This should be followed with a flush rinse of one quart of tap water. Door gasket should be checked for signs of wear.

2. <u>Transfer carriage</u>

   <u>Daily</u>: All accessible surfaces are to be washed with Calgonite solution, from the top downward. Casters should be cleaned last.

3. <u>Gas sterilizer</u>

   Refer to equipment operating instruction manual.

4. <u>Washer/sterilizers</u>

   Refer to equipment operating instruction manual.

Affected Departments

Reviewed _____

Subject	Effective Date 1-90	Latest Revision & Date
FOOD CART SCHEDULE		

Patient care floor personnel send carts containing patient food trays and utensils to decontamination via the soiled cart lift.

The carts are sent on a scheduled basis, approximately one (1) hour after the meal has been served.

Breakfast trays are returned at approximately 8:45A.M. Lunch trays are returned at approximately 12:15P.M. Dinner trays are returned at approximately 6P.M.

When the carts arrive in decontamination, they are noted on the decontamination log and moved to the dish machine area.

Dishes and utensils are processed in the dish machine. These have priority over the dishes from the cafeteria.

Carts are processed through the cart washer and returned to dietary immediately by dispatch personnel. They are used for the next meal.

Affected Departments

Reviewed _____

Subject	Effective Date	Latest Revision & Date
CART WASHING	1-90	

All carts are washed on a scheduled basis in one of the following ways:

1. In the automatic cart washer
2. By hand
3. By the Mikro spray unit and steam gun

Carts that are used to transport soiled items are washed after <u>each use</u>. These include trash carts, surgical case carts, and food tray carts.

Carts used for transporting clean supplies only are washed at least every six (6) months or as needed.

Affected Departments

Reviewed _____

Subject		Effective Date 1-90	Latest Revision & Date
SILVERWARE WASHING			

Silverware is stripped from the tray and placed in the soak tubs for 15 minutes.

After soaking, the silverware is removed from the soak tub, sorted, and placed in the silverware racks provided. All silverware must be placed in these racks by type: all knives together, all forks together, and all spoons together.

The racks are then loaded onto the conveyor and processed by the dish machine.

The racks are removed from the dish machine on the clean end by dietary personnel. If any silverware must be rewashed, dietary will notify materials management and pass the racks through the doorway to the dish machine area in decontamination.

Silverware is rewashed by hand, where necessary, and sent through the dish machine again.

Affected Departments

Reviewed _____

Page 1 of 1

Subject	Effective Date	Latest Revision & Date
DISH MACHINE AREA CLEANING	1-90	

The entire area around the dish machine and the dish machine itself are cleaned at the end of each day, after all items have been processed.

This includes: the dish machine (see the equipment operating instruction manual), the walls and the floors around the machine, the conveyors, and any external surfaces of the scraping station, etc.

A combination of cleanser, Staphene, the Mikro spray unit, and the steam gun are used.

The daily cleaning is the responsibility of the evening dish machine operators.

The daytime operators clean the area or the machine, as necessary, during use.

Affected Departments

Reviewed _____

Page 1 of 1

Subject		Effective Date 1-90	Latest Revision & Date
	UTENSIL WASHING		

Materials management receives soiled, used utensils, pots, and pans from dietary to be washed.

Dietary delivers these items to the dish machine area in decontamination via a cart. The cart is passed through the doorway adjoining materials management and the kitchen.

All utensils, pots, and pans will have been rinsed and soaked <u>before</u> presenting them to materials management.

Materials management transports the utensils to the triple sink area in decontamination, via the cart, for scrubbing/washing. They are placed on the same cart to drain.

After the items are clean, they are transported to the dish machine area and fed through the dish machine as a batch. Dietary unloads on the clean side (in the kitchen).

Any items requiring recleaning will be brought to the attention of materials management by dietary and returned to the cleaning area.

The cart used to transport the utensils, pots, and pans is processed through the cart washer and then returned to the kitchen.

Affected Departments

Reviewed _____

Subject	Effective Date	Latest Revision & Date
CLEAN DISH INSPECTION	1-90	

Dietary personnel inspect all items as they emerge from the dish machine, after processing. This is done in the kitchen area.

If any items are still not clean, they will be reprocessed, as necessary, by materials management.

Dietary accumulates these items on a cart and periodically pushes the cart into decontamination.

Materials management reprocesses the items, washes the carts, and returns them to dietary.

Any recurring problems are brought to the attention of the materials management manager in that area.

Affected Departments

Reviewed _____

SECTION XV

PATIENT TRANSPORTATION
SECTION XV

Subject		Effective Date 1-90	Latest Revision & Date
PATIENT TRANSPORTATION OVERVIEW			

Materials management/transportation is responsible for the timely, safe, and efficient transport of patients throughout the hospital. This is a centralized service for the entire facility.

All patients, even if ambulatory, will be escorted by a transporter or a nurse, if medical conditions require such attention and continuous medical supervision or care.

Patient transportation services are provided from 6:30A.M. to 7:30P.M., Monday through Friday, and from 6:30A.M. to 3:00P.M. on Saturday and Sunday. After hours, departments will provide their own transportation of patients.

Affected Departments

Reviewed _____

Subject	Effective Date 1-90	Latest Revision & Date
REQUESTS FOR PATIENT TRANSPORT SERVICE		

The dispatch office of materials management is the home base for patient transporters. The dispatcher assigns patient moves to transporters as requests are received.

Departments obtain patient transport service through two primary methods:

1. The master schedule that is developed every 24 hours includes all in-patient care services that require patient movement.

   a. The schedule displays the location, destination, and any unique transport requirements (IV pole, oxygen tank holder, extra large wheelchair) by time of day.

   b. The dispatcher assigns transport appointments so that patients arrive up to 10 minutes before the scheduled time.

2. Requests are received on an as-needed basis via telephone or computer message.

All requests are logged and handled on a first come, first served basis unless designated otherwise by the requesting department.

Any questions of priority are referred to the manager.

As staffing permits, transporters will respond to on-demand requests within 10 minutes of the time the request is received in dispatch.

When response time cannot meet this objective, the dispatcher notifies the requesting departments and attempts to reschedule or uses other materials management personnel to handle the patient transport.

Affected Departments

Reviewed _____

PATIENT TRANSPORTATION LOG

TIME OF REQUEST	DISPATCHER	CALLER'S NAME	PATIENT NAME	ROOM #	LOCATION (FROM)	DESTINATION	DUE TIME	TRANSPORT MODE (WHEELCHAIR, STRETCHER) REQUIRED

Subject			Effective Date 1-90	Latest Revision & Date
PATIENT TRANSPORT—PICKUP AND ARRIVAL				

On arrival at the patient location, the transporter will check in with the department receptionist and sign out the patient on the log (noting the time). Patients will not be transported without recording the movement on the log. This ensures that the patient's location is known to the patient care staff at all times.

In case of delays of more than 5 minutes in picking up a patient, the transporter will call the dispatch office to advise of the delay. Then, the transporter will report the delay to and request assistance from the department supervisor on duty to get the patient ready to move.

If there is a delay of longer than 8 minutes, the transporter will advise the receptionist that this transport should be reordered, and then will call the dispatcher for a new assignment. If there is no other assignment that takes a higher priority, the transporter will wait until the patient is ready.

On arrival at the destination, the transporter checks in at the receptionist's desk and completes the log, noting the time of arrival. The transporter remains with the patient until department personnel officially take charge of the patient. Any delays of more than 5 minutes are reported to the dispatcher.

Affected Departments

Reviewed _____

Subject	Effective Date	Latest Revision & Date
PATIENT HANDLING	1-90	

Patient transporters are thoroughly trained to handle patients in a manner that is effective and safe for both the patient and the transporter.

Departments requesting patient transport are expected to advise the dispatcher of the appropriate transport mode:
1. Wheelchair
2. Stretcher
3. Bed
4. Specialty mechanism

If the patient weighs over 200 pounds, two transporters will be dispatched or the transporter will obtain assistance from patient care staff. (This procedure is not necessary if the patient is fully ambulatory.)

Affected Departments

Reviewed _____

Subject	Effective Date	Latest Revision & Date
PATIENT RELATIONS	1-90	

Transporters are trained in and expected to use proper care techniques and etiquette when dealing with patients at all times. This goes beyond being courteous to an expression of true concern for the patient's well-being.

Transporters should pay close attention to the patient's condition (ability to move into the wheelchair, expressions of pain, etc.) and report these observations to the patient care staff on arrival at the destination or before departing if the patient seems to be in extreme distress. The transporter will follow the instructions of the patient care professional in charge regarding any change in handling methods.

If any problems arise or if a patient complains or is injured, an incident report must be completed within one (1) hour of the occurrence and reviewed with the director of materials management and the safety director.

Affected Departments

Reviewed _____

Subject	Effective Date	Latest Revision & Date
TRANSPORTER/DISPATCH COMMUNICATIONS	1-90	

Transporters will check in with the dispatcher via telephone, immediately following completion of a transport transaction to advise dispatch that the assignment has been completed and to obtain a new assignment.

Transporters carry pocket pagers so that the dispatcher can contact them to advise of cancellations, schedule or patient condition changes, etc.

Transporters should not return to the home base (office) before calling the dispatcher to see if there is a new assignment.

Affected Departments

Reviewed _____

Page 1 of 1

Subject	Effective Date 1-90	Latest Revision & Date
TRANSPORTATION EQUIPMENT		

All patient transport equipment is the responsibility of the transport department. This includes wheelchairs, stretchers, and special apparatus.

Equipment is maintained in both a central area adjacent to the dispatch office and decentrally at key user departments, which include:

1. Surgery/recovery
2. Physical therapy
3. Radiology

Three times daily (10A.M., 2P.M., and 6P.M.) transporters who are not moving patients will collect equipment and return it to designated location(s) so that it will be available for future transactions.

All transport equipment is cleaned by transport personnel, as needed and on a scheduled basis every 90 days, in the equipment cleaning area of materials management/processing. Records are maintained to make sure all equipment is cleaned according to the schedule.

Affected Departments

Reviewed _____

Subject	Effective Date	Latest Revision & Date
TRANSPORTATION RECORDS	1-90	

When a transportation request is received by the dispatcher, it is logged, noting the date, time, patient name, transport mode, and source/destination.

In addition, each transporter completes a patient transportation transaction record form for each move made. The information is identical to the dispatch information, plus:
1. A notation of the time the transaction was completed
2. Any notation of delay because the patient was not ready, patient release was delayed, or a patient care staff member was unavailable to help move the patient

The data is compiled daily, weekly, and monthly and is used by management to assess:
1. Workload volume
2. Service/response time
3. Productivity
4. Required schedule changes
5. Other problems or issues

Affected Departments

Reviewed _____

Subject	Effective Date 1-90	Latest Revision & Date
TRANSPORTATION RECORDS (cont.)		

PATIENT TRANSPORT TRANSACTION RECORD

Date _____   Transporter's initials _____

Patient name _____   Room # _____

Time request received _____   A.M. P.M.

Destination due time _____   A.M. P.M.

Time arrived to pickup _____   A.M. P.M.

Time arrived at destination _____   A.M. P.M.

Delay code (circle one or more)

1. Elevators
2. Patient not ready
3. Equipment not available
4. Second transporter required
5. Schedule error

Transport mode (circle one)

1. Wheelchair
2. Wheelchair with IV pole
3. Stretcher
4. Stretcher with rolling equipment
5. Ambulatory
6. Ambulatory with rolling equipment

Affected Departments

Reviewed _____

Subject	Effective Date 1-90	Latest Revision & Date
VERTICAL TRANSPORT—ELEVATORS		

Patient transportation and escorting both take place on the patient service elevators. Even ambulatory escorts do not use the public elevators.

When transporting patients in an emergency, transporters use the emergency access code to call the elevator. Emergencies take priority over all other transport requests.

When the emergency transport is completed, the elevator is released so it can return to the normal operating mode.

Affected Departments

Reviewed _____

SECTION XVI

WASTE HANDLING
SECTION XVI

Subject		Effective Date	Latest Revision & Date
	OVERVIEW	1-90	

While waste management is not a responsibility of materials management, waste <u>handling</u> is a key concern for <u>all</u> departments and staff members.

Materials management is also involved in many facets of storing or handling waste:

1. Sterile processing personnel remove waste from surgery via case carts.
2. Receiving dock personnel coordinate waste pickup with a hauler.
3. Dispatch personnel transport bulk trash collected on carts via the cart lift and/or service elevator to the lower level, then ultimately to the dock/compactor.
4. Materials management and/or housekeeping staff remove trash and accumulate it in the soiled utility room.

The institution adheres to federal, state, and local regulations regarding the handling of each type of waste. The categories of waste include:

1. Routine
2. Regulated/infectious/hazardous
3. Sharps
4. Radioactive
5. Chemical
6. Recyclable

Definitions of these categories are covered in the pertinent legislation and/or in the American Hospital Association guidelines.

Waste is handled so that patients, visitors, and staff are protected at all times.

Housekeeping maintains records of all waste transactions, according to the appropriate regulations.

Affected Departments

Reviewed _____

Page 1 of 1

Subject		Effective Date 1-90	Latest Revision & Date
ROUTINE WASTE			

Routine waste includes all materials that are not regulated; they have no hazardous properties. This includes trash, refuse, garbage, and any materials that do not require special processing or disposition.

Routine waste is handled as follows:

1. Waste is placed in clear poly bags at the location where it is generated.

2. Caution must be exercised at all times to make sure other waste categories are separated from routine waste.

3. Bagged waste is transported to the chute/tube system for movement to the ground-floor compactor located at the dock.

4. Trash that is too large to fit in the chute system is transported by housekeeping on a cart via the cart lift or service elevator to the ground floor and taken to the compactor by dispatch personnel.

5. Staff members should wash their hands immediately following handling waste or pushing waste-filled carts.

6. When the compactor is full (according to the indicator gauge), housekeeping contacts the hauler to remove the container and replace it with an empty container. During this exchange period, the trash chute/tube system is deactivated.

7. Carts used to transport waste are cleaned after each use in the automatic cart washer in decontamination.

Affected Departments

Reviewed _____

Subject	Effective Date	Latest Revision & Date
REGULATED/INFECTIOUS WASTE	1-90	

Regulated waste includes any material that is considered infectious and hazardous. It is defined by federal, state, and local regulations.

Regulated waste is placed in <u>red</u> poly bags and held in a separate cart in the soiled utility room.

1. When the cart is full, or at the scheduled times (10A.M., 3P.M., 8P.M.), the cart is sent via the cart lift to the ground floor.

2. Dispatch staff transport the cart to the regulated-waste holding room at the dock.

3. Daily, the regulated waste is picked up by a contractor and transported to an approved incinerator. Housekeeping personnel supervise this procedure.

4. The regulated-waste holding room is thoroughly cleaned by housekeeping.

5. Carts used to transport waste are cleaned after each use in the automatic cart washer in decontamination.

Affected Departments

Reviewed _____

Subject		Effective Date 1-90	Latest Revision & Date
	SHARPS		

Sharps include needles, glass ampules, syringes, and other materials that may puncture poly bags and injure/contaminate staff members. Sharps are considered regulated waste materials.

All sharps are placed in approved containers at the point of use. Containers are designed to avoid poke-through and injury.

Containers are collected, when full, transported by housekeeping personnel to the soiled utility room, and placed in trash carts with the regulated waste.

Regulated-waste carts are transported by housekeeping via the cart lift or service elevator to the ground floor. Then, dispatch moves the carts to the dock, where the waste is stored until picked up by the contractor.

When the full containers are collected, new containers are placed at the point of use by housekeeping staff. Containers are provided by materials management on the supply carts.

Affected Departments

Reviewed _____

Subject	Effective Date	Latest Revision & Date
RADIOACTIVE WASTE	1-90	

Radioactive waste is generated in nuclear medicine, radiation therapy, radiology, and research laboratories. It is placed in special containers at the point of use by personnel of the user department.

When containers have been filled, they are sealed, dated, and transported by department staff to the holding room at the dock.

To avoid the high cost of processing/transporting radioactive waste, it is stored until the radioactivity decays and the waste becomes harmless. This period is 140 days.

When filled containers are delivered to that room, all other containers are inspected. If the decay date has been reached, containers are placed in the compactor by department staff.

Affected Departments

Reviewed _____

Page 1 of 1

Subject	Effective Date 1-90	Latest Revision & Date
CHEMICAL WASTE		

Chemical waste includes dangerous waste generated by laboratories or the pharmacy (chemotherapeutic drugs).

All chemical waste is contained and taken to the chemical-waste holding room at the dock by personnel of the user department.

Three times per week (Monday, Wednesday, Friday), a contractor picks up all accumulated waste.

Housekeeping staff members complete all documentation after making sure that all waste being removed has been properly listed on the records.

Affected Departments

Reviewed _____

Subject	Effective Date	Latest Revision & Date
RECYCLABLE WASTE	1-90	

State and local waste regulations require sorting and recycling of the following materials:

1. Glass
   a. Clear
   b. Colored

2. Plastic
   a. Clear
   b. Colored

3. Aluminum, metal

4. Corrugated cardboard

5. Paper

Recyclable material is sorted at the point of use by personnel of the user department and placed in a container designated for each type of material.

Filled containers are transported to the soiled utility room by housekeeping staff for transport via the cart lift or service elevators to the holding room at the ground floor/dock area.

On Thursday, or as needed, the materials are picked up by the city hauler or contractor, depending upon the type of material. Housekeeping staff maintain records of all transactions.

Affected Departments

Reviewed _____

Page 1 of 1

ABOUT THE AUTHOR

Active in the healthcare industry since 1972, Jamie C. Kowalski specializes in the area of operations management. Consulting engagements have included operations auditing; the analysis, planning, and implementation of operational and computer systems; facility planning; capital equipment planning and budgeting; feasibility and cost/benefit studies for shared services development and for contract versus in-house support services; and strategic and marketing planning projects.

Kowalski has experience as a director of materials management and assistant vice-president for support and general services in community and tertiary hospitals. He has also managed and marketed a computerized materials management system and hospital consulting service for a national hospital supply manufacturer/distributor.

He has authored articles in several industry journals and was a contributing author in *Cost Containment in Hospitals* and *The Handbook of Health Care Material Management*, both published by Aspen Systems. An editorial board member of a national professional journal, he is a frequent speaker at seminar programs.

Kowalski has achieved member status in the American Association for Health Care Consulting and the American College of Healthcare Executives, fellow status in the American Society for Hospital Materials Management, and is a certified professional (CPHM) by the Health Care Materials Management Society. He earned both an MBA and a BS degree in business administration at Marquette University, Milwaukee, where he was elected to the Beta Gamma Sigma Academic Honor Society.